IV VITAMIN REGULATIONS

YOUR GUIDE FOR USP 797 PHARMACY COMPLIANCE

SHANNON PETTERUTI, NP

COPYRIGHT

CONTENTS

To the Rhode Island Board of Pharmacy. For without your constable arriving, this book would have never been written.

And to my husband who processes information quickly.

WHY I WROTE THIS BOOK
FOR YOU

The aim of this book is to help you to understand how USP 797 impacts your group medical practice, health clinic, wellness center, med spa, or other health-related business that offers IV vitamin infusions. As an owner, manager, clinician, or other employee, it is vital that you understand how governmental enforcement of USP 797 can determine whether your healthcare-related business will be able to operate or be closed by governmental regulatory authorities. You probably are already aware that USP 797 can "make or break" your clinic or med spa offering IV infusions of any kind to people who depend upon your services. In turn, this may be causing you anxiety and sleepless nights. Or not, because you do not even comprehend the scope of USP 797 and its ramifications.

Like most people in your type of business, you also may not know how to deal with a federal or state inspection of your facility for USP 797 compliance. The good news is that you now have a way to learn the necessary information for your IV vitamin infusion-related business without wading through lengthy governmental documents written in legal language. In recognition of your likely hectic daily life and schedule, this "self-help" book is purposely concise while still packed with information you need to know.

After you take the Quiz in Chapter 1 of this book, the next two chapters provide background knowledge for you about USP 797, including how it came to exist and why governmental authorities (federal, state, and local regulatory entities) are so focused on enforcing it. Chapters 4 and 5 present infection control and safety "best practices" as related to the delivery of IV vitamin infusions. From Chapter 6 onward, this book is primarily devoted to helping you to prepare for an inspection for USP 797 compliance performed by a federal or state regulatory entity. Not only is preparing your wellness center or other healthcare business for inspections covered, but also how to deal with an inspector's determination of a deficiency in USP 797 compliance (whether or not this results in a citation or other legal action against you).

My goal in writing this book is for you is to enable your clinic or center offering IV vitamin infusions to maintain the highest level of USP 797 compliance such that you can "hold your own" if a regulatory authority chooses to inspect your center. This can be accomplished if your understanding of USP 797 is increased and you take the steps described in this book.

"Why should I believe what you say?" you may be asking yourself. This is the primary reason: through my years of experience opening vitamin infusion centers nationwide along with extensive research, I have been able to extract from the voluminous USP 797 documents those elements that are essential to the operation of IV vitamin infusion centers. Another reason is because I provided IV vitamin infusions in a health center, and was tremendously impacted by the enforcement of USP 797.

Unfortunately, a book like this one did not exist for me to read at that point in time, so I had to learn about the USP 797 enforcement implications by experiencing them first-hand. I truly do not want you to have to go through my miserable personal experience. Let me explain through telling you the following story.

MY JOURNEY INTO USP 797 COMPLIANCE

One perfectly normal day, to my complete shock, a Constable arrived at the center. I happened to be standing near our Medical Director when that Constable unexpectedly walked in and handed him a letter.

The normal day suddenly turned into a horrible one for us. I still clearly remember how the Constable asked our Medical Director – in a neutral but firm tone of voice – to open the letter. As required under the Law, the Constable remained standing next to him to witness our Medical Director read the letter (and those seconds felt like hours to me). This was how I came to learn that our highly-skilled and dedicated Medical Director of our IV infusion center had been legally "served."

In case you have never seen such a letter, it really is a heart-stopper. "SUMMARY SUSPENSION" was the letter's headline, and it ordered this physician to stop practicing medicine immediately. In other words, our Medical Director and our IV infusion center were considered to be imminent threats to the public.

Were we shocked? Yes, indeed. Did I ever expect such an occurrence? Not in my wildest dreams.

First of all, there had never been a single patient complaint. Secondly, there had not been any adverse outcomes. In fact, we had been providing IV vitamin infusions safely long before IV vitamin infusions began to attract popular attention (and years before the number of vitamin infusion centers across the US began to surge). In other words, we were an "early" provider of this type of outpatient health service.

Possibly our worst offense (in the eyes of our critics and governmental regulatory authorities) – that caused such extensive regulatory scrutiny to rain down upon us – was that our health center was so financially successful that it inspired others in our geographic area to open their own IV infusion centers. Whoever goes first in any industry is apt to receive far more scrutiny, even when it fills a healthcare service need. That was our unfortunate circumstance.

But, I had done my homework so thought we were sufficiently prepared. Given all the Hollywood celebrities touting the benefits of IV vitamin infusions and consequent mass media interest, I knew our health center (and especially because of its success) would eventually attract governmental regulatory attention. Therefore, I made it my business to have us operate at the highest possible infection control, patient safety, and regulatory compliance level.

In order to accomplish this, I researched everything that I could find about how to safely run an IV infusion center. While I was aware of USP 797, my information sources contained discrepancies as to how it might be applied to an outpatient IV vitamin infusion center. This is because USP 797 guidelines had been developed for compounding pharmacies and not centers like ours. After all, the USP 797 guidelines had been developed before outpatient IV vitamin centers like ours even existed. Nevertheless, I realized that USP 797 could be applicable to our health center, so made it my business to ensure that our center adhered to it.

"What did I do to ensure adherence?" you may wonder.

The abbreviated answer to this question is that I purchased a high-quality isolation hood (the exact one used in our local hospital) for mixing the vitamins. I ensured that our center had medical-grade refrigeration equipment. I only ordered supplies from 503B-designated compounding pharmacies. Basically, I did everything I could think of (and everything I could research). At that time, I believed that I had taken every necessary step to make sure that our IV infusion center would not only be positioned to provide the highest quality service to patients, but also withstand any regulatory scrutiny from state agencies.

Our patients loved us, and they were thriving with our treatments. However, the medical establishment did not understand what we accomplished for our patients, so did not approve of what we were offering in this "new" healthcare arena. Likewise, the state Board of Pharmacy inspectors did not know what to make of us as a healthcare business.

Do you remember the old cliché: "The most important things to learn are the things you learn after you thought you knew everything?" This is what I learned from my first-hand experience at that time. Since then, I have become well aware of the reality that IV vitamin infusion centers have opened without regard to either USP 797 or a recognition of the paramount importance of sterile technique. Their sloppiness – and especially in practicing sterile technique – has consequences for those of us who do embrace IV vitamin infusion "best practices" and adhere to governmental regulations.

No wonder that regulatory inspections of IV infusion centers have been exponentially increasing across the country, and becoming something that all IV vitamin infusion centers are likely to undergo!

After our Medical Director received that suspension letter, I determined to learn everything I could about USP 797 compliance, so that what happened to our Medical Director would not happen again. Over time, I became an expert in USP 797 protocols. Moreover, I worked closely with pharmacists who were involved in the creation of those protocols. Like most government regulatory documents, USP 797 as a document is enormous, confusing, and (in some aspects) conflicted. The challenge for me was determining what applied to IV vitamin infusion centers, and ascertaining how to apply it in a way that would not be so costly as to result in the loss of the business through bankruptcy.

Meanwhile, there were other infusion centers in my community that began to reach out to me for guidance in complying with USP 797. One center was preparing to undergo a renovation estimated at $500,000 in order to meet USP 797 requirements, until I was able to show them a less expensive way to achieve compliance.

Fortunately, our IV vitamin infusion center survived regulatory oversight and our Medical Director has his license reinstated. Looking back at that time, I can understand what motivated the Board of Pharmacy to take the actions that they did against our health center. It really is the responsibility of those of us who choose to innovate in the healthcare realm to ensure safety. Furthermore, it is our responsibility to be aware of the local, state, and federal regulations that we must follow.

I am always grateful for hardships that teach me important lessons. This was certainly the case with that phase of my professional life as a clinician and business owner, as I had no choice but to become one of the nation's leading experts in how to apply USP 797 to IV infusion centers.

The takeaway for you from this story is that – despite facing dismaying regulatory hurdles– I was not only able to ensure the survival of our health center, but used the knowledge and experience acquired to subsequently become co-founder of an IV vitamin infusion center franchise, *THE DRIPBaR*. In my CEO role and co-founder at *THE DRIPBaR*, I have had the opportunity to travel across the US to both open new *DRIPBaR* centers and learn about the competition. What is apparent is that the vast majority of infusion centers are out of compliance with USP 797.

Do not despair. Your business offering IV vitamin infusions can be successful while achieving local, state, and federal regulatory compliance. It is time now to dive into the complex subject of this "self-help" book and get started on your journey toward understanding USP 797 compliance!

1

TAKE THIS QUIZ!

The questions below require "yes" or "no" answers.

1. Does your IV Infusion Center have specific assignment of quality functional responsibilities as defined in a Quality Assurance plan?
2. Does your IV Infusion Center have an independent Quality Systems Department whose responsibility is to ensure that the facility, equipment and personnel meet the demanding standards set forth by the United States *Pharmacopeia* (USP)?
3. Is your IV Infusion Center committed to and in compliance with USP 797 guidelines for sterile compounding?
4. *(Two-part question)* Are all significant procedures performed in the IV Infusion Center covered by Standard Operating Procedures (SOPs)? Is there documentation that the IV Infusion Center staff has been trained and understand the SOPs?
5. Is your IV Infusion Center's Quality Assurance plan reviewed both annually and whenever changes are made to the plan?

6. Does your IV Infusion Center's facility meet or exceed USP guidelines for compounding pharmacies?
7. Does your IV Infusion Center have separate areas dedicated to performing sterile and non-sterile compounding, product inspections, labeling, raw material storage, and dispensing?
8. Is the air quality in your IV Infusion Center engineered for HEPA filtration to reduce particulates?
9. Does your IV Infusion Center conduct tests of air and surface samples of your clean room and other controlled environments?
10. Does your IV Infusion Center perform and document daily, weekly, and quarterly cleaning to assure a clean and safe facility?
11. Is your IV Infusion Center's staff properly trained to perform aseptic manipulation skills, gowning technique, clean room use, and successfully perform media fills on a yearly basis?
12. Does your IV Infusion Center's staff take steps to minimize error and maximize the prescriber's intent for the patient during the compounding process?
13. Does your IV Infusion Center purchase pharmaceutical-grade chemicals (USP, NF equivalent) from *FDA*-registered suppliers?
14. Does your IV Infusion Center perform post-filtration filter-integrity testing?
15. Does your IV Infusion Center have systems in place for handling complaints and investigating sterility failures and adverse events?

(**Important Note:** If you answer "no" to any of the following questions, you are not in compliance with USP 797, and need to take action to attain compliance in order to prevent dire consequences as a result of a local, state, or federal regulatory inspection of your health clinic, wellness center, or other health-related business. If you answer "yes" to everything you still may not be in compliance with YOUR state board of pharmacy. Be sure to look your states specific guidelines).

2

WHAT IS USP 797?

You may already know that the *Food and Drug Administration* (*FDA*) is a federal agency within the US *Department of Health and Human Services* that regulates medications and vitamin supplements. While the *FDA* enforces regulations pertaining to a business like yours that provides vitamin infusions to people by an intravenous (IV) route, the US *Pharmacopeia* – an independent nonprofit – sets standards for them. Chapter 797 of the US *Pharmacopeia*'s monograph of standards pertains to sterile medication compounding.

"What does this have to do with my clinic, physician practice, wellness center, or business?" you may wonder. The answer is "everything" if you do not want to experience the disastrous ramifications of not complying with those standards in offering IV vitamin infusions. While a different US *Pharmacopeia* (USP) monograph chapter – USP 795 – is focused on non-sterile compounding, the one that is the focus of this booklet is concerned with *sterile* compounding.

You may be scratching your head right now because you – as the owner, operator, manager, or clinician in a business offering IV vitamin infusions – do not see yourself as compounding anything. You are definitely not alone in this belief. If you are currently puzzled as to why you need to familiarize yourself with USP 797 (rather than just leave this to your attorneys or legal department), it is because providing IV vitamin infusions is not only viewed as pharmaceutical compounding, but considered *sterile* compounding by all regulatory entities enforcing USP 797. Moreover, any of these diverse regulatory entities can wreak havoc on your business if you are not in compliance with USP 797.

Here is the reason why offering IV vitamin infusions changes the regulatory oversight of your business to something far more extensive. Basically – unlike vitamins in pill form– the risk of infection is astronomically-increased when an IV is the method of vitamin delivery, because sticking a person's vein with a needle can cause bacteria and viruses to directly enter the bloodstream. As stated in USP 797, "Understanding the risks inherent in sterile compounding and incorporating established standards are essential for patient safety. Compounded medications made without the guidance of standards may be sub-potent, super potent or contaminated, exposing patients to significant risk of adverse events or even death.

In other words, you are now considered a compounding *pharmacy* – from a USP enforcement perspective – if you are offering IV vitamin infusions to your clients, patients, or customers!

It does not matter if you think your business (and the employees of your business) are knowledgeable in providing IV vitamin infusions and the recipients of these infusions are happy with them. Regulatory entities will make unannounced visits to check up on any business offering such infusions to ensure that USP 797 compliance is actually occurring.

News flash. The individuals sent by these regulatory entities are tasked with turning over every leaf to find evidence of noncompliance in order to protect the public. If no noncompliance is found, it might appear to their supervisors that these regulatory staff were derelict in their job duties! Therefore, their inspection role incentivizes these lower-level employees to find something wrong about your business operations to report back to their supervisors.

Most problematically for you, a report of some type of noncompliance can not only result in a legal citation but can completely shut your business! Therefore, you really do need to have a plan of action in place to ensure that you can do the following: 1) comply with USP 797; 2) prepare for both scheduled and unscheduled visits from the representatives of regulatory entities; and 3)cope with any citations for noncompliance with USP 797 should this occur.

This is why it is not enough for your attorneys or legal department to understand what to do to keep your business in compliance, but the institution of USP 797 compliance "best practices" needs to become a key component of managing your business on a daily basis.

CREATING A PROJECT MANAGEMENT FRAMEWORK FOR USP 797 COMPLIANCE

Just as project management plans typically include the diverse tasks necessary to accomplish the project, resources required to accomplish each of the identified tasks, number of needed employees, training, expected expenditures, and an internal evaluation process to ascertain whether the project is proceeding according to plan or needs some modification, a similar approach will be necessary for you to comprehend your basic capacity to be deemed "in compliance" with USP 797 by regulatory entities. In case you did not already guess this core element of simultaneously managing multiple projects within a business, an intensive level of documentation will be vital for ascertaining on a *daily basis* whether you are in compliance with USP 797 – so you can make immediate changes if you discover a compliance gap exists.

To comply with USP 797, compounding pharmacies need policies and procedures (also called Standard Operating Procedures [SOPs] or protocols) that cover specific situations that arise during compounding. For example, the following are a few of the areas that should be addressed (and that need to be incorporated into your project management framework for USP 797 compliance): 1) verification of accuracy and sterilization of every item utilized in the provision of IV vitamin infusions; 2) environmental quality and control of every part of your clinic/facility; 3) verification of automated compounding devices and related equipment; 4) final checks by staff prior to Compounded Sterile Products (CSP) release for use; 5)storage and Beyond-Use Dating (BUD) of each item; 6) proper processing in the specific compounding environment; 7)product quality control; and 8) patient/client monitoring and adverse effects reporting.

The US *Occupational Safety and Health Administration* (*OSHA*) expects hospitals to engage in infection control implementation, and an Infection Control Coordinator who is a Registered Nurse (RN) is the employee who typically oversees this implementation and monitoring. Your outpatient healthcare practice, clinic, or wellness center – if you are "acting" as a compounding pharmacy by providing IV vitamin infusions – will need an employee assuming a similar role since patient (and staff) safety and infection control are foundational to compliance with USP 797.

Therefore, your project management framework with regard to the "project" of infection control needs to include the following subcategories: 1) engineering controls (such as the use of sterilizing equipment); 2)administrative controls (such as clear reporting authority); 3) safe work practices (including cleaning/disinfection processes and the handling of hazardous waste); 4)evaluation mechanisms to ascertain employee understanding – or lack of understanding – of safety and infection control practices; and 5)personal protective equipment or *PPE* (such as protocols related to the wearing of face-masks, gloves, and gowns, along with the overall plan for continuous *PPE* availability). Yes, there is a tremendous amount of overlap between infection control practices and sterile compounding "best practices" for the provision of IV vitamin infusions!

Of course, training – and intermittent re-training – of your employees (as well as tracking of your employees' understanding of what they have learned in the training sessions, and incorporation of the knowledge acquired from these trainings into daily practices) is also critical to USP 797 compliance. Regulating entities that send representatives to evaluate your compliance will most likely want to see documented evidence of such training.

If you are already beginning to experience a headache, this is a sign that your project management framework and/or project plans are not as detailed as they should be when it comes to being fully-prepared to meet the USP 797 compliance requirements of regulatory entities. It cannot be emphasized enough that creating detailed SOPs/protocols for every step in the various processes involved in providing people who seek IV vitamin infusions from your business with such infusions is essential. After all, you do not want your clinic or practice to be featured on TV *News* or on the Internet for causing preventable harm!

There is yet another key point related to project plans/SOPs before we can move on to another topic. Expecting people to utilize technology (such as cloud-based technology) to view your carefully created protocols is not enough. You need to have them written down and available to anyone who needs to see them – so binders with printouts of all your protocols are strongly recommended. Besides the possibility that there could be a computer problem the day a representative of a regulatory entity shows up at your door (which could cause that employee to cite you for USP 797 noncompliance), the following paragraph describes other reasons for not maintaining solely computer-based SOPs/protocols requiring access to a networked computer.

Employees of regulatory entities may want to review certain SOPs/protocols to determine your USP 797 compliance with specific aspects of USP 797. If these protocols are only viewable on computer systems that contain a database with *HIPAA*-protected information about your patients/clients (and/or a database of personnel information about your employees) – this could create a "Catch-22" for you in terms of compliance with different types of regulatory entities that could cause your business to be legally-cited for a violation or permanently shuttered.

7

DEMONSTRATING CORE COMPETENCIES

Besides project management activities crucial to USP 797 compliance (and regulatory entity assessment of that compliance), a key takeaway from this chapter is to recognize the necessity of being able to show core competencies to regulatory entities in the following arenas that are discussed in detail in later chapters: 1) hand hygiene; 2) garbing; 3) cleaning and disinfection; 4)calculations, measuring, and mixing; 5) aseptic technique; 6) achieving and/or maintaining sterility; 7) use of equipment; 8) documentation of the actual compounding process for every item compounded; and 9) adherence to "best practices" in the movement of materials and personnel within the compounding area (as well as the entire physical area of your clinic or practice).

The other foremost takeaway from this chapter is that the enforcement of USP 797 occurs via federal, state, and local regulatory entities. The *FDA* is a federal entity, but a Department of Public Health or Department of Pharmacy is a state entity (as are many licensing Boards). Local health boards may also exert some authority over your business, as well. These entities all have different requirements to validate your USP 797 compliance – and some even have conflicting requirements. Yikes!

However, to truly comprehend why the oversight of IV vitamin infusion-offering businesses is expanding to such a degree, it is important to understand how *and* why these regulations came into existence. Likewise, it is also important to understand some upcoming (or probable) regulatory changes in order to prepare for them. The history of compounding pharmacies is why your business – no matter how much your patients and clients depend upon your services and recommend them – is likely to come under intensive regulatory scrutiny if you are offering IV infusions.

It is now time for you to begin your journey into IV infusion regulatory history as presented in the next chapter.

KEY TAKEAWAYS FROM THIS CHAPTER

- USP 797 is the US *Pharmacopeia*'s "best practices" guidance document for sterile pharmaceutical compounding that is enforceable by governmental regulatory authorities such as state Boards of Pharmacy and the US *Food and Drug Administration* (*FDA*).
- If you provide IV vitamin infusions at your health clinic or other health-related business, your facility is considered a sterile compounding pharmacy for the purposes of USP 797 regulatory oversight.
- To comply with USP 797, you need to develop policies, protocols and Standard Operating Procedures (SOPs) and be able to demonstrate adherence to these SOPs upon regulatory inspection.

3

HISTORY OF COMPOUNDING PHARMACIES AND THE LEGAL LANDSCAPE

The American public was outraged when – in 2012 – a steroid medication injected into the spine to treat back pain caused a widespread fungal infection affecting more than 750 people across the US and resulting in 64 deaths. The *New England Compounding Center* (*NECC*) – a compounding pharmacy located in Framingham, MA – was found to be in violation of its state pharmacy license, as well as the former USP 797 regulations existent at that time. Besides a major fine and closure, its owner was sentenced to years in prison. This is the backdrop to the exponential increase in federal and state regulations governing the operations of compounding pharmacies that now impacts all outpatient settings providing IV vitamin infusions.

However, numerous prior periodic incidents of preventable fatalities caused by infections resulting from injected medications led to the initial creation of USP 797 in 2004. This chapter in the US *Pharmacopeia*'s book of standards was aimed at medications compounded outside of a controlled manufacturing environment for prescription medications. Since then, the USP 797 has been revised twice (in 2008 and 2019).

Although the US *Food and Drug Administration* (*FDA*) was created in 1906 and oversees prescription drug manufacturing, it has never regulated medications and vitamins created in compounding pharmacies. In contrast, the *FDA* regulations (besides governing the approval process for prescription medications prior to public availability) are aimed at (GMPs) of medications by drug manufacturers. Notably, these GMPs are inclusive of the methods, facilities, and controls used in the manufacturing, processing, and packing of any given drug product. (When current GMPs as opposed to previous GMPs are referenced in *FDA* guidance documents, they are referred to as cGMPs.)

It actually took the creation of USP 797 by the US *Pharmacopeia* – which sets standards for governmental regulatory entities – for the *FDA* to be able to enforce this practice standard focused on the sterile compounding of injectable medications. State pharmacy departments, the *Joint Commission on Accreditation of Healthcare Organizations* (*JCAHO*), and other state licensing boards also rely on USP 797 in their licensure and regulatory decisions related to compounding pharmacies (inclusive of IV infusion providers). Without a state license, compounding pharmacies cannot operate at all. State rules applicable to compounding IV infusions (including IV vitamin infusions) are updated periodically, and commonly under the jurisdiction of individual state Boards of Pharmacy – which operate in all 50 states.

Meanwhile, the US *Food, Drug, and Cosmetic Act* (*FDCA*) was enacted in 1938 granting the *FDA* with specific regulatory authority. Subsequently, the US Congress passed the *Drug Quality and Security Act* (*DQSA*) in 2013 in order to grant additional oversight to the *FDA* (with Title 1 of *DQSA* specifically pertaining to compounding). There were two *DQSA* Title 1 parts applicable to sterile medication compounding; these were Section 503A and Section 503B.

This is a "heads up" moment as outpatient IV vitamin-infusing sites are often confused as to which Section is applicable to them when they purchase vitamin infusions for use in their site. In a nutshell, Section 503A created a "safe harbor" for traditional pharmacy compounding performed for a specific patient prescription (such as occurs in hospitals or in the satellite clinics of hospitals); this means the compounding pharmacies covered by Section 503A are generally overseen by state Boards of Pharmacy without *FDA* involvement unless a patient complaint has been legally filed.

Furthermore, *FDA* oversight is not as intensive under Section 503A (except when a legal complaint has been filed) as under Section 503B – which is the section applicable to "outsourcing" facilities for compounded medications (inclusive of vitamin infusion contents). Under Section 503B, a pharmaceutical compounder can voluntarily register on an annual basis with the *FDA* as an "outsourcing facility." While an outsourcing facility must adhere to cGMP, that facility does not need to receive *FDA* approval for its compounded products prior to the marketing of its products.

Yet, this creates a dilemma for centers providing IV vitamin infusions where infusion packages/products are purchased from an "outsourcing facility." USP 797 requires the use of a 503B pharmacy rather than a 503A pharmacy. Meanwhile, 503A pharmacies have not traditionally been held to the same regulatory adherence level in terms of "best practices" as 503B pharmacies. This means that a vendor producing the infusion packages/packets that you utilize who is found noncompliant of USP 797 upon regulatory inspection can lead to your health center or clinic also being determined noncompliant.

Hear Ye! If you are an outpatient physician practice, naturopathic clinic, wellness center, or other independent business providing IV vitamin infusions, you really need to be careful about which "outsourcing" compounder you choose to acquire your products. This is because choosing one that is not recognized by pharmacy departments and the *FDA* as engaging in cGMP could be held against you and considered a USP 797 violation during an inspection by regulatory employees. Not to mention cause potential harm to your patients, employees, and overall business!

503A VERSUS 503B COMPOUNDING PHARMACIES – A COMPARISON OF REGULATORY REQUIREMENTS

One of the foremost differences between 503A and 503B facilities (and a major component of cGMP) is the requirement for every process to be validated in a 503B facility. In other words – before any new product can be brought to market – multiple batches must be made and submitted for both testing and stability studies to ensure the given product's safety. While this can result in a longer time needed to get new products to customers, it ensures that every batch made during normal production is consistent in quality, and meets the standards set by the *FDA* and according to cGMP.

Not only must the products be validated, but – in accordance with USP standards – testing methods must also be validated so as to ensure accuracy and precision. Furthermore, all vendors that supply raw materials must be thoroughly vetted, and with on-site inspections performed by the Quality Assurance team for all critical suppliers.

For better comprehension of this important issue affecting your ability to achieve USP 797 compliance, the following table illustrates some of the regulatory differences between 503A compounding pharmacies (which are generally found in hospital settings) and 503B compounding pharmacies. Specifically, this table compares regulatory requirements between 503A and 503B within the classifications of: 1) regulatory governance; 2) environmental monitoring; 3) product labeling, 4) required quality assurance system, 5) finished product dating, 6) bulk drug substances, and 7) registrations, as follows:

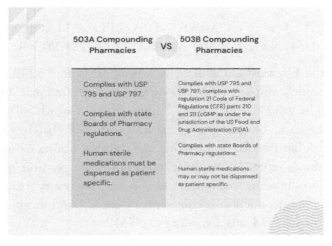

Regulatory Governance

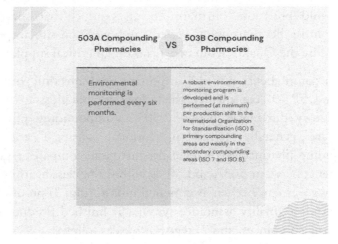

Environmental Monitoring

503A Compounding Pharmacies	VS	503B Compounding Pharmacies
Patient information, medication information, company information, and adequate directions for use of medication.		Labeling requirements per the US Drug Quality and Security Act (DQSA).

Product Labeling

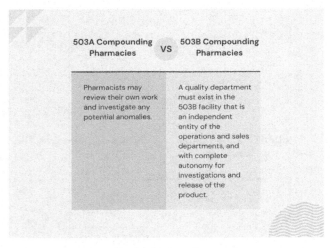

Quality Assurance System

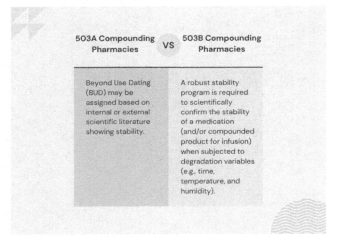

Finished Product Dating

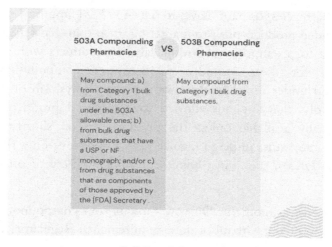

Bulk Drug Substances

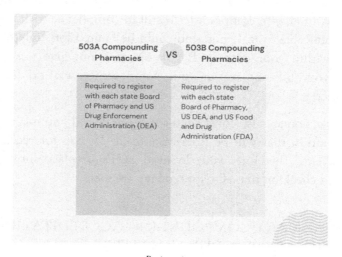

Registrations

MORE THINGS TO REMEMBER ABOUT 503B COMPOUNDERS THAT CAN IMPACT YOUR HEALTH CLINIC

The following are five other things to bear in mind in relation to the use of compounding pharmacies as suppliers of infusion packages/products to your health clinic or health-related business. Firstly,

503B pharmacies do not have to receive *FDA* approval for their compounded products prior to marketing them (plus have the capacity to qualify for exemptions regarding labeling products with adequate directions for use). Secondly, 503B-covered compounders must compound under the supervision of a licensed physician or pharmacist, Thirdly, they are not allowed to compound products already commercially available unless the products are on shortage status. Fourthly, they must undergo regular *FDA* inspections on a risk-based schedule. Fifthly, they must adhere to a wide variety of other regulations.

Let's pause for a moment. Do you know if your compounding pharmacy is complying with all of these requirements? Regulatory authorities expect you to know! Therefore – as a business that is providing IV vitamin infusions – you really need to always stay current with whether your chosen compounder is still in compliance with the regulations applicable to it. If not, you could be faulted for something not actually within your control. Regulators may not give *you* a "pass" because you did not realize your compounder was no longer in compliance.

Meanwhile, you are also considered a compounder if you mix anything into a solution that will be inserted into an IV bag for receipt by a patient/client. Therefore, you do need SOPs in place for regularly performed checking that all requirements are met.

THE PHARMACY COMPOUNDING ACCREDITATION BOARD (PCAB) AND WHY IT MATTERS

The *Pharmacy Compounding Accreditation Board* (*PCAB*) – a voluntary standard for compounding pharmacies – was established shortly after the initial creation of USP 797. *PCAB* was formed by eight national pharmacy organizations (including the US *Pharmacopeia*), to serve as a voluntary accrediting body for the practice of pharmacy compounding.[v] Since *PCAB*-accredited compounding pharmacies are limited to those that successfully meet *PCAB*'s requirements, you are more likely to be dealing with a reputable compounder if it has this designation.

USP 797 REVISIONS IN 2007 AND 2019

In 2007, revision to the USP 797 allowed several exemptions/exceptions to building full clean rooms by outpatient centers providing IV infusions (since the original USP 797 targeted solely compounding pharmacies). This was due to resistance by centers providing IV infusions as consequent to the high cost of building full-scale – but unnecessary at that scale – clean rooms.

Until 2019, the US *Pharmacopeia* designated three levels of risk as it related to compounded pharmaceuticals: low, medium, and high – with the risk level based on assessment of the compounding environment. At that time, the focus was changed to an emphasis on *where* the compounded preparation was being made rather than the determination of a specific risk level of low, medium, or high. This occurred in order to clarify for outpatient centers their real level of compounding risk, so as to eliminate their high frustration when trying to achieve *FDA* rules compliance.

Other USP 797 changes in 2019 pertained to personnel qualifications and pharmacy facility requirements. The changes to personnel qualifications are especially important for businesses providing IV vitamin infusions, in that training related to the need for sterile compounding is extended to all employees and not simply the employees who are compounders. In other words, all personnel (including housekeeping and other non-clinical staff members) accessing compounding areas must demonstrate competency in proper behavior to maintain the required environment.

Additionally, a person was required as of 2019 to be designated as the responsible employee to ensure that anyone entering the sterile compounding area could maintain its sterile environmental quality. Moreover, another responsibility ascribed to this management-level employee through this USP 797 change is that conduction of the daily operations of the sterile compounding area are occurring in accordance with USP 797 standards.

Meanwhile, one of the major changes in terms of pharmacy facility requirements was that CAI/CACI systems are now called Restricted Access Barrier Systems (or RABS) and they must be placed in the clean room suite to get Category 2 BUDs. A clean room "suite" consists of at least two rooms: an anteroom and a buffer room.

Yet other 2019 changes pertained to air and surface sampling; Beyond Use Dates (BUDs); aseptic sterilization versus terminal sterilization; compliance with master formulation requirements; and pharmacy quality assurance and control.

PROPOSED USP 797 REVISIONS FOR 2022

In September 2021, proposed changes to the USP 797 were issued to be effective in 2022. The most significant proposed change is the inclusion of Category 3 compounded sterile preparations (CSPs). This new category would be in addition to the Category 1 and 2 CSPs that were in the previous revision in 2019. The addition of Category 3 involves significant changes in how pharmacies compounding CSPs must operate if identified as falling within Category 3.

These categories are linked to specific requirements related to Beyond Use Dates (BUDs). For example, Category 1 CSPs are compounded under the least controlled environmental conditions and therefore are assigned a BUD of 12 hours or less (plus other specified requirements). The proposed revision state that Category 3 sterile preparations can have longer BUDs compared to those for Category 1 and Category 2. However – in order for these longer BUDs to apply – the Category 3 sterile preparations have a number of additional requirements specified beyond that associated with Category 2 preparations.

(This change is the result of some regulators discovering that expired compounded pharmaceuticals were still being utilized in the treatment of patients. Therefore, you need to ensure SOPs related to checking the BUDs of all of your supplies used in the provision of IV vitamin infusions.)

There really is no way to get around the need for you to do your "homework." It is generally considered your responsibility to keep abreast of the upcoming USP 797 changes. Since these have not been finalized, further description of the proposed revision is not included in this chapter. On the other hand, the only thing for certain is that changes will occur.

Attitudes toward preventing avoidable infections have shifted toward an increased willingness by healthcare facilities and providers to shift away from usual standard protocols to far stricter ones in consequence of the Covid-19 pandemic. Indeed, the Covid-19 pandemic has necessitated even tighter scrutiny on the part of businesses providing IV vitamin infusions upon their safety and infection control practices. Although this really has nothing to do with USP 797, the increased federal and state governmental focus on infection control due to the Covid-19 pandemic means that even more scrutiny is likely to occur upon inspections by regulatory employees tasked with ensuring adherence to USP 797 than prior to the onset of this coronavirus pandemic.

Therefore, the next two chapters are targeted at overall "best practices" for infection control so contamination by an infectious agent (*pathogen*) – whether bacteria, virus, fungi, or parasite – does not transmit to a recipient of an IV vitamin infusion at your facility. We will begin with a focus on IV infusion "best practices" as linked to infection control since the correct usage of IV apparatus is central to providing an IV vitamin infusion.

KEY TAKEAWAYS FROM THIS CHAPTER

- Strict regulating by governmental authorities in accordance with USP 797 was the historical consequence of a lack of adequate adherence to current Good Manufacturing Practices (cGMP) at compounding pharmacies resulting in patient deaths.
- Compliance with USP 797 requires that you utilize a 503B

compounding pharmacy rather than a 503A compounding pharmacy.

- If you provide IV infusions at your health center or other health-related business, using a 503B pharmacy as your supplier that is not in compliance with USP 797 could be considered as a USP 797 violation by your health-related business upon regulatory inspection.

4

INFECTION CONTROL: FOCUS ON OVERALL "BEST PRACTICES"

Preventing infection in both your patients and staff is paramount to your business reputation. People receiving IV vitamin infusions want to maintain or improve their health – not worsen it through contracting an infection. Nothing can do more to make the employees of regulatory entities suspicious of your ability to comply with USP 797 than a history of infections linked to your healthcare center or facility. As you probably know all too well, bad publicity about your center due to an infection outbreak can take a major toll on your business' ability to survive (as well as attract the negative attention of your state's Department of Public Health, Department of Pharmacy, and various licensing boards.

Not only the wearing of gloves and gowns when manipulating any part of the IV apparatus (such as bag, tubing, or needle) is important to reducing the chance of enabling a pathogen to be transmitted into a clinician or recipient's bloodstream, but adherence to all nursing sterile procedure "best practices." (Please note that you will need to maintain documents that contain your sterile procedure SOPs so that both clinicians and their paraprofessional healthcare support staff can quickly locate them to review these SOPs as necessary.)

In recognition that you might not be a clinician yourself, it bears repeating that every part of the IV apparatus (and not just the insertable needle) needs to be used following clinical sterile procedure "best practices," so that the vitamin-infused solution that will drip through the tubing into a patient's vein does not become contaminated by a pathogen (*e.g.,* bacteria) during any step of the infusion process.

Likewise, a staff member who has an infection can potentially transmit that infection to other employees as well as patients. Therefore, sick staff members who work with patients should not be in the workplace – and a protocol needs to be in place to require that they not come into the workplace when ill. Guess what? In order for this infection control measure to be followed, all of your personnel (or Human Resources Department) employees need to understand that infection control as "workplace culture" is imperative for your business to remain "open."

BACTERIA TRANSMITTED BY CONTAMINATED IV APPARATUS AS CAUSE OF INFECTIONS

The three most common bacterial contaminants are *Staphylococcus*, *Pseudomonas*, and *Klebsiella*, but the foremost bacteria as a contaminant is *Staphylococcus aureus* (often termed *Staph. aureus*). Although skin infections with *Staph. aureus* are far more common than blood infections, a blood infection with *Staph. aureus* can cause death (besides infecting internal organs such as the heart, lungs, and kidneys).

Since so many people who seek IV vitamin infusions have weakened immune systems (such as consequent to recent chemotherapy treatments for cancer or a genetically caused vitamin deficiency), contracting any type of infection can be even more life-threatening for them. Therefore, the key takeaway of this paragraph is understanding that an infection contracted during a visit to your clinic or wellness center can be especially dangerous for the patients/clients most likely to *need* IV vitamin infusions to improve their health. Therefore, your facility needs to be even more careful in terms of prioritizing infection control.

The Hippocratic Oath for physicians is "First, do not harm." It is my strong belief that this equally applies to your business or outpatient clinical practice providing IV vitamin infusions.

PROPER HANDWASHING AS ESSENTIAL FOR INFECTION CONTROL

Your staff need to comprehend that handwashing with an antibacterial soap between caring for each patient/client (and especially if providing the actual IV vitamin infusion) is absolutely foundational to infection control. Likewise, they need to understand that if a staff member has a bacterial infection on the skin, this can be easily transmitted to all other staff and patients. Therefore, it is essential to ensure that your staff and patients understand (and engage in) "best practices" pertaining to hand-washing *and* proper hand-washing technique.

The following is essentially the *Center for Disease Control* (*CDC*)'s five-step protocol for proper handwashing:

Step 1:

Wet hands with clean, running water (warm or cold), turn off the tap (using a paper towel so as not to touch the sink spigots with the hands), and apply soap to hands.

Step 2:

Lather hands by rubbing them together with the soap. Besides lathering the palms, lather the backs of hands, and between fingers, and under the nails.

Step 3:

Scrub hands together for at least 20 seconds.

Step 4:

Rinsehands well under clean, hot, running water.

Step 5:

Dry hands using a clean paper towel or air dry them (without touching the installed air dryer).

Your staff also need to understand that utilizing an alcohol-based hand-sanitizing product between caring for patients is not an acceptable replacement from an infection control standpoint to washing hands with soap and water. Hand-sanitizing products are better than nothing, but cannot clean hands to the same level as washing them with soap and water. Therefore, you need to have an SOP in place to ensure that proper hand-hygiene is actually occurring – and especially among any staff provide direct care to your patients/clients.

Of course – for this to occur – you need to have SOPs in place to ensure that the plumbing supplying hot water is working satisfactorily; every product needed for staff to easily perform hand-hygiene is continuously-stocked at optimal levels; and that there are no obstacles to performing this extremely *basic* infection control at your clinic or center. Likewise, cleaning of both compounding and patient care areas needs to occur on a frequent basis at pre-scheduled times, as well as documentation of all cleaning/disinfecting episodes. This all may sound very elemental to you, but – all too often – the elemental aspects of infection control during a busy day in a workplace can be neglected by staff members under pressure!

As you may already be aware, staff can become so busy that they do not perform proper hand-hygiene prior to performing IV vitamin infusions. The bad result can be an infection in a patient or staff member that you will need to document as an "adverse event" – and then explain upon regulatory inspection if the representative of the regulatory entity requests more information as to how the infection was contracted. The more "adverse events" due to poor infection control practices, the more likely that your clinic or center will be required to undergo an inspection from a regulatory entity.

KEY TAKEAWAYS FROM THIS CHAPTER

- Infection control is essential to preserving public perceptions of the overall safety of your health clinic or med spa and your business reputation.
- Proper hand hygiene is essential to preventing the spread of infectious agents from one patient who is receiving an IV vitamin infusion to another at your health center *as well as* between employees at your health center.
- Outbreaks of infection at your health center or other health-related business increase the likelihood of USP 797 regulatory inspections and scrutiny by local, state, and federal regulatory authorities.

5
INFECTION CONTROL: FOCUS ON IV INFUSION "BEST PRACTICES"

L et us now consider the intravenous (IV) preparation room. Obviously, the room in which compounded sterile products (CSPs) containing IV nutrients are prepared should not enable anything to occur that could cause contamination by a pathogen of anything in the room and/or the acquisition or transmission of an infection. However, not all your employees (or external repair personnel) enabled entry to this area may actually comprehend the need to always follow infection control "best practices" when inside this room. For this reason, you will need detailed (and documented) safety and infection control protocols related to *anything* that occurs in this room. Even the floor, walls, and door to it!

As previously mentioned, is crucial to recognize that USP 797 considers your clinic or center to be a "compounding" site. This is especially the case in terms of your IV preparation room and related storage areas. Therefore – besides implementation by your clinicians of pertinent infection control measures (such as the wearing of facemasks, gloves, and gowns) – regulatory employees will expect compliance with the requirements for safety and infection control as contained in USP 797.

Please pause for a moment and take a deep breath. While adhering to the requirements in USP 797 may seem to you not applicable to what your clinic or center that offers IV vitamin infusions is doing on a daily basis, *not* following these requirements contained in USP 797 can result in a regulatory citation or worse!

In order to comply with USP 797, the following standards for your IV preparation room need to be met. Firstly, it needs to have adequate lighting. Secondly, it needs to have a specific level of ventilation (and with air filters replaced once every two months). The entire area needs to be cleaned on a regular basis (but at least weekly), and with all surfaces wiped from higher to lower in the room. New (disposable) *non-woven* cleaning cloths need to be used when wiping countertops used in IV preparation (as well as any containers that hold syringes or needles). It is also essential to have a sink in this room for hand-washing (in order to enable proper hand-hygiene) – and that arena for handwashing needs to be at least five feet away from your compounding isolator/hood.

You may think this sounds simple enough (if you have such a room). However, your staff needs to understand every step of the written protocols addressing this room. This means that each and every staff member that is allowed to enter this room needs to understand your protocols, so a lot of training will be required. Who can enter the room – and who is not allowed to enter it – needs to be clear to every person in your center's site. Likewise, the handling of anything not in the protocol (such as the finding of an empty cup of coffee in the IV preparation or the accidental spilling of a solution on the floor) needs to have a documented protocol, as well as monitoring for compliance with the protocols (inclusive of specific infection control protocols).

EXAMPLES OF ITEMS REQUIRING DOCUMENTATION OF CLEANING/DISINFECTING IN A LOG:

Staff need to document the following specific cleaning/disinfecting occurrence within the sterile compounding area on a daily basis to achieve compliance with USP 797: 1)compounding isolator/hood; 2) all horizontal surfaces; 3) high touch surfaces; 4) all floors; and 5) emptying trash.

Meanwhile, staff need to document on a monthly (plus everyday) basis – besides all parts of the compounding isolator/hood – the following to remain in compliance with USP 797: 1) all surfaces of ceiling; 2) walls and all surfaces pass-through; 3) all surfaces of furniture, trash bins, outside surfaces of Primary Engineering Controls (PECs); and 4) all storage bins and shelves.

Solely on a monthly basis, the following need to receive cleaning/disinfecting: 1) general "prep area"; 2) refrigerators/freezers; 3) centrifuge; and 4) anything else located in the sterile compounding area (*e.g.,* fan blades). Of course, the name of the person who performed the cleaning/disinfection and date/time this occurred need to be included in the documentation.

"BEST PRACTICES" RESULTING FROM THE COVID-19 PANDEMIC:

The current Covid-19 pandemic means that infection control measures aimed at *respiratory* infection control need to be implemented, besides the other infection control "best practices" – so you need to bear this in mind while reading the rest of this chapter, which includes ideas conceived before the Covid-19 pandemic commenced. Now let us proceed to discuss cleaning/disinfecting in far more detail.

CLEANING/DISINFECTION AND OTHER IV-RELATED "BEST PRACTICES" – NOT AS CLEAR AS IT MAY FIRST SEEM FOR REGULATORY ADHERENCE

As noted in Colleen Huber's online book, *Best Practices Guidelines for IV Preparation* (which pertains to "best practices" but is not focused on compliance with USP 797 requirements), the counter top for IV preparation needs to be a non-porous surface, and all countertops should be wiped down with a new, clean, wet cloth. I need to add at this point – due to the USP 797 requirement pertaining to cleaning/disinfection – that your non-woven cleaning cloth (or wipe) needs to be *low-linting*, as well. If not, your health clinic could be considered not in compliance with USP 797 by a regulatory inspector.

Huber's book additionally notes that the cleaning cloth should be dried thoroughly at the end of every workday, and personnel working over the countertop cannot sneeze, cough, sigh, or even speak while working over the counter or any injectables.

But wait. There is more to consider. If a person performing the IV preparation speaks to someone, that person should back slightly away from the work area, or twist 90 degrees to speak to someone else so as to not face the injectables. In the event of a cough or a sneeze, the above-referenced book suggests turning 180 degrees away, stepping away from the counter, and sneezing into one's bent elbow – and then changing the gloves or washing the hands again.

(Consequent to the ongoing Covid-19 pandemic, please note that it also makes sense that a facemask, gloves, and gown be worn, and that all personnel be vaccinated against Covid-19.)

Furthermore, Huber's book states:

"Needles and syringes used in IV preparation are kept in clean closed containers. They stay in their original manufactured packaging until the moment of use. Nothing enters those containers, at any time, whether solid, liquid or gas, that may compromise the sterility of the needles and syringes used in IV preparation.

Refrigerated injectables must be maintained at a temperature of 34 to 38 degrees Fahrenheit, until ready for use. The refrigerator is inside the IV preparation room. Again, no food or drink, or human specimens share the refrigerator with sterile injectables. Those injectables are kept in a dedicated refrigerator. The injectables are organized and clearly labelled, so that there is no more handling of them than necessary.

Vials of sterile liquids remain closed at all times and protected from room air. These vials should be stored in dedicated cabinets or drawers at room temperature, or in the dedicated refrigerator, as directed by the manufacturer, at all times except when needed for use."

Including this description is really just to emphasize how important detailed protocols are for preserving "sterile conditions" in the room where the IV vitamin infusion is being prepared. The reality is that bacterial contamination can easily occur due to suboptimal protocols of infection control. Then, the bacteria can grow and contaminate everything with which they come in contact. Not only will that make the cleaning and disinfection process that much harder, but it can make both employees and patients sick. Therefore, good infection control practices (including the cleaning and disinfection practices) have to be carried out at all times and *documented*. This is the area that a regulatory employee is sure to inspect carefully.

Most of all, nobody in your clinic or center should be involved in compounding anything that will enter the body of a patient who is not licensed and clinically trained in that capacity. That is a sure-fire way to ensure that your clinic or center will be shut down by a state and/or federal regulatory authority.

KEY TAKEAWAYS FROM THIS CHAPTER

- Inspectors from regulatory authorities such as state Boards of Pharmacy and the US *Food and Drug Administration* (*FDA*) will expect – and scrutinize for – compliance with requirements for safety and infection control as contained in USP 797.
- Nothing in the room in which compounded sterile products (CSPs) containing IV nutrients are prepared should enable contamination by an infectious pathogen to occur, and SOPs pertaining to activities in that room need to reflect this adherence to sterile processes for infection control and safety.
- Employees of your health clinic or other health-related business who enter the room in which IV nutrients are prepared need to understand every step of the SOPs addressing activities in this room, along with all requirements for documentation of their activities. Consequently, a related plan of action for the training of employees is necessary.

6

PREPARING FOR CONTACT BY A GOVERNMENT REGULATORY AUTHORITY

Most of the time, regulatory inspectors do not forewarn you and just arrive without any advance notice at your health center. However, it is possible (though not as probable) that you may receive a letter that your clinic or center will receive an inspection by regulatory employees of a federal, state, or local regulatory authority. That notification letter or unexpected visit by a regulatory inspector will most likely emanate from your state's Department of Pharmacy (also known as Board of Pharmacy) simply because it considers your business – as one that offers IV vitamin infusions – a compounding pharmacy! Furthermore, it is likely to request some specific documentation from you (that is assumed to be in your records).

Whether you receive a letter of notification or an unexpected visit by a regulatory inspection team depends on your state regulators' customary practices and the particular circumstances. However, it is likely that you will not receive any advance notice from the *FDA* or even your state's Department of Public Health if there was a complaint or adverse event associated with your health clinic, med spa, or wellness center. This is why you absolutely need to be prepared at all times for an inspection by all of these regulatory entities (as well as clinical licensing boards).

Notably, state-legislated *Acts* provide inspectors from state Departments of Pharmacy with the legal authority to inspect any business designated a "pharmacy" to ensure that these are meeting minimum legal standards of operation and practice as defined by applicable state and federal laws. Regulatory staff members from Departments of Pharmacy *routinely* inspect pharmacies (and especially compounding pharmacies) for various reasons, including the granting of requested permitting/licensing; inspection after receipt of request for change of location or change of ownership; cyclically-scheduled inspections for compliance; and federal/state enforcement activity.

Due to the greatest likelihood that the requestor for completion and return of enclosed forms – inclusive of the written statement of notification for your clinic or center to receive an inspection for compliance with USP 797 – will be your state's Department of Pharmacy, this is the starting-point for this chapter.

PREPARING FOR A DEPARTMENT OF PHARMACY DECISION TO INSPECT YOUR CENTER

It cannot be overstated that all Department of Pharmacy requests by regulatory staff members for copies of documents should be answered immediately. However, there is a high probability – if the number or scope of requested documentation is large – that additional time to provide all the documents will be granted upon request. State pharmacy departments typically must legally-allow a realistic and sensible window for the provision of these records (and especially if these are solely maintained electronically and need to be "printed out"). It is common practice by many centers to provide a written response that you will comply with the provision as soon as possible, and that you will have the copies for them inside of the legally mandated window.

The day you are first approached by the Department of Pharmacy (such as by an inspector conducting a "surprise" inspection visit) is the day that you need to alert your legal department or contact your lawyer. (If your business lawyer is not experienced in interacting with governmental regulatory entities and their staff, you need a lawyer that does understand how to deal with them in order to avoid even more regulatory interference in your day-to-day operations.)

If an inspector sees something amiss, that inspector is likely to immediately require closure of your IV vitamin infusion center – even if only temporarily. Obviously, this can be very damaging to your reputation and business.

While implementing a project management plan, embracing "best practices" in safety and infection control, and careful documentation is metaphorically your clinic's *Department of Homeland Security*, coordinating a response to the request for documentation (plus a future inspection visit) can be a collaboration of your Department of Homeland Security, your legal department, and all management-level employees and/or clinicians overseeing patient safety and infection control. This is your *Department of Defense*!

This is absolutely essential for you to remember:

Once an inspector arrives from the Department of Pharmacy, the time is long past to think about preparation.

Therefore, it cannot be emphasized enough how important documentation of your SOPs and everything else matters at this point. Your electronic and "print" manuals, SOPs, training materials, completed checklists, completed forms (and templates of forms), and all other documentation will represent your clinic's daily practice to the inspectors.

If you have this extensive level of documentation, you can take a break to meditate and calm yourself. This is going to go a long way to demonstrating compliance motivation to potential inspectors!

PREPARING FOR A SCHEDULED DEPARTMENT OF PHARMACY INSPECTION

It is an excellent idea to create a "compliance" binder that contains – besides other content such as core SOPs – the following: 1) copy of license issued to your health center by your state's Department of Pharmacy; 2) any out-of-state licenses or permits linked to your health center; 3)copy of US *Drug Enforcement Administration* (*DEA*) permit if your center has one; 4)clean room certifications; and 5) any other paperwork (such as specific completed forms that are dated and signed) routinely requested by regulatory inspectors.

It is also important to be aware that there are legal limits to access by inspectors to your center's physical facility (including its compounding area), offices, and records. It is vital that you know these legal limits, as you can better comprehend how to tactfully decline if inspectors request viewing something that is not legally-allowable under your state's laws applicable to its Department of Pharmacy. Yes, you should meet with your lawyer to familiarize yourself with what is allowable and what is not!

All suggestions, comments, or interactions with an inspector should be written down for your (and your lawyer's) records. This is jumping ahead, but – as mentioned in an article in *Pharmacy Purchasing and Products* magazine – it is important to resist the urge to make any immediate changes to your center's operations during the inspection to satisfy an inspector's request. This is because – similar to determining the best project management framework for you before finalizing it for implementation – a broad plan of corrective action requires careful considerations and planning (and should not be undertaken until after that inspection has concluded). This will allow the plan to reflect input from "experts" and "best practices," while also simultaneously accounting for all of the downstream issues that changes to your compounding room operations and other health clinic arenas may cause.

This is an added tip. To manage a regulatory inspection effectively, adherence to your advance- created written policies and procedures (which can be classified as a tentative project within your project management framework with its own staff and resources linked to it) is key. This lessens the need for you to improvise – and potentially improvise badly when you need to "impress"!

Indeed, once an inspector arrives at your business for an inspection, the time is long past to think about preparatory steps. My key point here is that prior planning will reduce the potential for confusion leading to a lengthier inspection *and* suspicion of noncompliance by inspectors.

SUGGESTED LIST OF PREPARATORY ACTIONS

Rather than wait until you feel that a bomb has just dropped on your healthcare practice, clinic, or wellness center, the following is a list of suggested actions for you to take to prepare for a Department of Pharmacy inspection (as noted in an article published in the *Journal of Health Care Compliance*):

1. Keep a record of all communications with State Boards of Pharmacy.
2. Organize all records into an inspection binder and ensure that the "pharmacy" (your health center!) is not missing any important documents.
3. Prepare staff so they know what to expect (inclusive of both training and practice "drills").
4. Ensure the "pharmacy" is clean (utilizing proper cleaning and disinfecting procedures and products).
5. Ensure that the medication refrigerator and other equipment are correctly-operating (and not operating in a manner other than the intended purpose, such as for storage of staff food items).
6. Ensure that any expired, recalled, or damaged/altered medications (*e.g.,* vitamin vials) are stored correctly or destroyed.

THE IMPORTANCE OF DESIGNATING A KEY EMPLOYEE TO ENSURE INSPECTION PREPARATION

It is definitely advisable to identify one employee to field questions from a regulatory inspector during the visit to your center. In this way, you can avoid conflicting information provided to that inspector that could raise that visitor's suspicions about your clinic not being in full compliance. After all, if different employees are providing different answers (even though the answers are essentially saying the same thing), it can appear that "one end does not know what the other end is doing" at your health center.

To avoid this type of miscommunication, identifying one specific employee for this role (and an "understudy" in case that employee is absent from work on the day of the inspection!) will both minimize disruptions and ensure that the responses are consistent with your clinic's policies and procedures addressing inspections. My recommendation is that the designated employee be a Registered Nurse (RN) or other clinician holding a current clinical license – as well as a management-level employee of your clinic. This is because a non-clinician (such as a front-desk worker) may not be able to respond to questions in as knowledgeable a manner and confuse scientific terminology in speaking without realizing the error in order to immediately correct it.

It is essential that this designated employee understands the limitations on the breadth and scope of regulatory authority, and be familiar with all policies, procedures, and protocols at the health center. Key tip: if this employee is unavailable when the inspector shows up at your clinic, suggest to that inspector that – from the inspection vantage point – things will proceed in a more efficient and organized fashion if the inspector is willing to return when the designated employee is available. My suggestion is that you state this with diplomacy but confidence and firmness, so that you are more likely to acquire agreement. If the inspector says "no," only then allow the "understudy" for the absent designated employee to perform this role.

PREPARING FOR AN FDA DECISION TO INSPECT YOUR CENTER

Please bear in mind that the following describes something far less likely to occur than an unexpected *FDA* inspection with no advance notification. However, notification may occur in some rare instances. Overall – while it is far more likely that you will be contacted by a state regulatory authority for documentation or the scheduling of an inspection – you may also be contacted as described in the previous section on contact by the Department of Pharmacy from a federal regulatory employee of the *Food and Drug Administration* (*FDA*). As previously stated, this is most likely to occur as the result of a patient's complaint or an adverse event occurrence at your clinic. (An adverse event does not need to be your clinic's fault, and can include an accidental staff needle-stick as well as a patient's allergic reaction to an injected nutrient.) On the other hand, the increased scrutiny of compounding pharmacies combined with exponential nationwide growth in IV infusion centers (including IV vitamin infusion centers) is leading to ever-increasing *FDA* notice.

One of the differences impacting preparing for an *FDA* inspection is that – in contrast to a state regulatory entity – the *FDA* is far less likely to schedule the inspection date *with* you. Instead, they are more likely not to notify you of the date. This means that you are less able to pick a less-hectic date than might otherwise be possible (or one that does not conflict with your vacation plans). As you may already be well aware from experience in attempting to contact a federal agency for a different reason, it can also take a great deal more time to speak to a member of a federal regulatory agency's inspection team even if you are provided with a phone number. There is significant understaffing among the federal workforce due to congressional actions that annually-constrain their hiring budgets. Therefore, do prepare to be on "hold" for a long time!

PREPARING FOR A DEPARTMENT OF PUBLIC HEALTH DECISION TO INSPECT YOUR CENTER

Your state Department of Public Health (DPH) may decide to inspect your center if a patient or client acquires an infection from receipt an IV vitamin infusion at your clinic. Likewise, a DPH inspection may occur as the result of an infectious outbreak linked to your clinic. Of course, a Covid-19 "cluster" linked to your facility is sure to result in a visit by DPH inspectors. Similar to a request for documentation by the Department of Pharmacy, a request for documents and the scheduling of an inspection by the DPH is a serious matter that requires immediate action by you. While it is unlikely that the US *Center for Disease Control* (*CDC*) will become actively involved in the inspection by the DPH, infections are federally reportable by the *DPH* to the *CDC*. Therefore, you can bet that – if the DPH becomes involved – your clinic will become scrutinized for state and federal regulatory compliance for years to come!

KEY TAKEAWAYS FROM THIS CHAPTER

- Regulatory authorities rarely warn you in advance of an inspection, and instead the inspectors nearly always show up at your health center without any advance notice to you.
- You need to be prepared at all times for an inspection of your health clinic or other health-related business for compliance with USP 797 by inspectors from regulatory authorities such as a state Department of Pharmacy or US *Food and Drug Administration* (*FDA*).
- Once a regulatory inspector arrives at your med spa or other health-related business, it is way past time to think about preparing for an inspection such as by maintaining required documentation. Failure to prepare in advance can result in dire consequences for you such as the closure of your med spa or other health-related business.

7
TRAINING (AND RE-TRAINING) YOUR EMPLOYEES

No doubt if you an owner or perform a marketing role in an outpatient practice, clinic, or wellness center offering IV infusions that you already fully aware that employee actions matter when it comes to your reputation with patients and clients. Maybe you have a personnel department or solely one employee acting in a human resources management role. One of the categories in a project management framework (as well as a business plan) is human resources. Even if you are a physician in a solo practice, your practice most likely includes a nurse and receptionist.

A project management approach requires that you think about the following. How many employees do you have (and how many do you need to function at a level that you can comply with USP 797 requirements)? What qualifications, background, training, licensure(s), and other factors are required of each employee role existent in your center? What employees can be subcontractors rather than actual employees of your business? What are the policies, protocols, and SOPs for hiring, training, and firing your employees? Obviously, these are just some of the decisions that will need to be delineated by you and/or your team into policies linked to the on-the-job functioning of your employees. Although clinicians typically are required to obtain a minimum number of Continuing Education Units (CEUs) through attending in-person or online courses, there is much on-the-job training that occurs for clinicians. Never mind every other employee of your clinic or wellness center.

According to an online article dated October 23, 2014, "Staff training is one of the most important parts of the USP 797 guidelines because personnel errors are often a problem with CSPs [Compounding Specialized Pharmacies]. Over a period of about two years, the *FDA* conducted 150 inspections at facilities that prepare CSPs. In 90 percent of these inspections, they found objectionable conditions, which were typically safety and sanitary problems. Some examples: workers wore soiled gloves, technicians wiped their faces, and staff didn't change gloves while preparing CSPs."

This article continues by suggesting the following six training tips to help your staff maintaining UPS 797 compliance:

1. **Perform a thorough gap analysis**. Following a determination of your CSP risk level, perform a current gap analysis to determine your current compliance level with USP 797 by comparing your pharmacy's current procedures with USP 797 guidelines.
2. **Emphasize personnel cleaning and garbing order**. In other words, emphasize safety and infection control! Basically, proper attention to safety and infection control will go a long way to ensuring compliance. My recommendation is that your center holds required training (and periodic re-training) sessions to query staff about their cleaning and garbing practices. Likewise, make sure they know the order for donning their personal protective equipment (PPE).
3. **Teach and reinforce proper hand-washing techniques.** (Utilizing a combination of verbal instructions, PowerPoint slides, and video is more effective than solely one type of method.) This was covered in an earlier chapter, so you now know how to do it!
4. **Teach staff correct documentation procedures.** To prove

compliance, everyone involved in CSP preparation must document all tasks performed; the documentation must clearly identify and explain what procedures were followed. However, that is not enough for demonstrating USP 797 compliance to regulatory authorities. Every employee role in a setting where IV vitamin infusions occur really is linked to some type of documentation in order to have a safe environment – with infection control as an essential component of that safety. When a clinical or non-clinical employee, demonstrating an understanding of SOPs and documentation procedures is critical to avoiding USP 797 noncompliance.

5. **Make sure staff are evaluated on key procedures.** It is not enough to train (and re-train) staff. They must also be evaluated and tested on an ongoing basis to assure that they have absorbed the information provided in trainings. If a deficiency in comprehension in a staff member is determined, that staff member must undergo re-training and then, a reevaluation. (Conducting evaluations will be covered in detail in a later chapter.) The reality is – for the sake of your compliance capacity – only employees who can demonstrate that they understand the information provided in their trainings can be allowed to perform the given procedures. An incompetent employee can cause you to become noncompliant, so that employee may sadly not be the right "fit" for their workplace! When it comes to any environment that provides IV infusions, competence is crucial so *ensure employee competence.*

6. **Develop and implement a systemic competency evaluation system.** (This is covered in Chapters 11 and 12.)

EDUCATIONAL LEVEL OF YOUR STAFF AND ADAPTING TRAININGS

Some of your staff will hold at least a four-year college degree, while others may have a two-year degree or solely a high school diploma.

SHANNON PETTERUTI, NP

Meanwhile, some of your staff (and especially medical assistants such as aides and housekeepers) may not be native English-language speakers. Yet others may be fluent English speakers but have lesser fluency in reading and/or writing in English. For your clinical staff, some may have graduate degrees while others – performing the same roles – may not (and some may be currently-licensed while others are not yet licensed).

Nobody performing a role requiring an active clinical license should be performing such a role without licensure, but that is a separate issue. The key takeaway of this subsection is that the trainings need to be geared at the educational level and understanding of your employees or they are not going to learn the information in the trainings.

HOW MUCH TRAINING SHOULD YOU PROVIDE?

The short answer to this question is "enough training to ensure that your practice or center is in compliance with USP 797." Even more crucial is that they receive enough training to ensure safety/infection control; excellent provision of services to patients and clients; the performance of their roles embracing "best practices" for their roles; and preserving your clinic or wellness center's reputation as a reputable and "high-quality" provider of IV infusions.

This is Essential for You to Remember:

All new employees will need to undergo initial training to learn your applicable policies and SOPs. However, periodic re-training is often necessary as "best practices" sometimes change, and staff can forget what they have learned as time goes by.

This is especially possible if some employees – due to feeling under work pressure from co-workers or because of a lack of interest due to personal problems – fail to consistently adhere to "best practices" for safety and infection control. When nobody is looking, some employees will get sloppy. This happens in most work environments. However – in a setting where IV infusions are performed – that can lead to the

44

transmittal of an infection or an accident (such as incorrect attachment of tubing to an IV bag resulting in leakage or blockage).

Therefore, retraining of all employees needs to occur on a regularly-scheduled basis – and appropriate to the specific employee roles within your "compounding pharmacy." For you to be ready for a state or federal regulatory entity to conduct an inspection, you also need to make sure that all your employees are trained (and retrained) in documentation linked to their specific role. Likewise, it is also prudent to train employees what to do if they notice a failure of documentation by some other employee in a similar or different workplace role.

In case you were wondering about it, you do need a SOP for "failure to document" notifications by your employees. If no SOP exists, your employees may not know what they are expected to do upon spotting a documentation failure, and simply neglect to report it to a supervisor or you (which would allow the failure to be corrected). In case you have not guessed it by now, the potential ramification could be that a regulatory inspector is the person who first notices that particular documentation failure – resulting in a legal warning of noncompliance!

You may be worried at this moment about the lost productivity that will occur as the result of training (and retraining) your employees which can require an hour or more per session. However, the health and well-being of your patients and clients are at stake, and poorly-trained staff are far more likely to make health-affecting mistakes that can leave you vulnerable to a lawsuit. Additionally, responding to a Department of Pharmacy or *FDA* warning of USP 797 noncompliance or reputational damage to your healthcare center (such as lowered private insurers' quality rating and/or Medicare quality rating issued by the *Centers for Medicare and Medicaid Services* [*CMS*]) is really not worth the risk.

Now relax, please. With careful planning performed in collaboration with your personnel staff, management team, and clinicians, you can implement a realistic action plan for training and retraining your employees to meet USP 797 requirements.

KEY TAKEAWAYS FROM THIS CHAPTER

- Staff training is one of the crucial parts of ensuring USP 797 compliance because staff errors are a major contributor to infections among patients/staff and adverse events.
- Following a determination of your health center's risk level as a Compounding Specialized Pharmacy (CSP), it is critical to compare your current compliance level with USP 797 written guidelines to identify areas needing improvement *prior to the actual occurrence of a regulatory inspection.* This includes aspects of staff training that can affect the compliance capacity of your health center.
- All new employees will need to undergo initial training to learn your applicable policies and SOPs. However, periodic re-training is often necessary as "best practices" sometimes change over time, and staff can also forget what they have learned as time goes by.

8

WHEN THE FDA INSPECTS YOUR BUSINESS PROVIDING IV INFUSIONS: WHAT TO EXPECT

L et us switch gears to focus again on the problem of facing regulatory inspections. Since an *FDA* inspection of your clinic or wellness center will most likely occur without any advance notice (and cause immediate closure if any USP 797 compliance violation is identified), this chapter is focused on the *FDA* inspection process. Fasten your seatbelt, as compliance with your state's Department of Pharmacy regulations pertaining to USP 797 are not the same as the *FDA*'s requirements.

Before launching into a description of the *FDA* inspection process, there are two things you really need to memorize. While Departments of Pharmacy determine compliance based on USP standards plus state regulations, the *FDA* – besides USP standards – will determine your USP 797 compliance based on federal cGMP rules (which were the regulations intended for ensuring the safety, standardization, and quality of products by drug manufacturers for pharmaceutical companies). In other words, your clinic or wellness center that mixes vitamins into a solution and places this mixture into an IV bag (like any "compounding pharmacy") is viewed from an *FDA* regulatory standpoint as a drug *manufacturer*!

Meanwhile, it is also important to grasp that an *FDA* inspection is totally different than an inspection conducted for *International Standards Organization* (*ISO*) certification or as part of a surveillance audit (in case you are familiar with these due to your specific type of business).

The *FDA* website states the following regarding their compliance inspection procedures:

"FDA may conduct an inspection of your operation for a variety of reasons, such as a routinely scheduled investigation, a survey, or a response to a reported problem. The investigator will present credentials and "Notice of Inspection" (FDA Form 482) upon arriving at your plant. A knowledgeable person in your firm, such as the plant or production manager, preferably designated ahead of time, should accompany the investigator at all times. It is in your best interest to fully understand FDA's inspection procedures. When you are unsure of certain actions taken by the investigator, don't hesitate to ask questions.

Usually, the investigator will examine your production process, look at certain records and collect samples. At the conclusion of the inspection, the investigator will discuss with your firm's management any significant findings and concerns; and leave with your management a written report of any conditions or practices, which, in the investigator's judgment, indicate objectionable conditions, or practices. This list of "Inspectional Observations," also called an FDA Form 483, can be used by your firm's management as a guide for corrective action, since the FDA representative will not usually recommend specific corrective measures. Your firm can and should respond to the FDA-483 during the discussion with the investigator. In fact, corrective actions or procedural changes that were accomplished immediately in the presence of the investigator are regarded as positive indications of your concern and desire to voluntarily correct discrepancies.

If you do not agree with the actions being taken by the FDA or if you have a question about the jurisdiction of the agency in a particular matter, you can contact the FDA's Office of the Ombudsman to seek a resolution."

If only it were that simple and straightforward. However, you now realize that the process is far more complicated since any evidence to the regulatory investigators of something not performed as expected by them can lead to a negative outcome for you.

How your clinic or center presents itself when the *FDA* inspectors arrive will generally set the tone for the inspection. Organization and confidence will project a favorable impression, but keeping them waiting will project the opposite. Upon their arrival, escort them into a private office or room where employees except your designated team assembled for this purpose is present (per your project management framework and inspection "action plan"). In addition to the management representatives, your clinic should have a designated person – preferably from your Legal Department – present who will act as a "scribe" to take minutes of the meeting(s) that occur during the inspection and record all requests for documents and records requested by the inspectors.

However, you are not required to provide records of management reviews, internal audits, supplier evaluations, and financial data as these are considered confidential – and generally not required under federal law to be provided to the inspectors.

FIRST STAGE OF THE INSPECTION VISIT

At the beginning of the inspection, ask the inspectors if they would like to view a PowerPoint or video presentation about your clinic – and suggest that this will assist them in better understanding how your clinic functions. This is not only an excellent opportunity to show off your employees' (and clinic's) competence in providing care to your patients/clients but can provide an overview of how your clinic (and its Quality Management System [QMS] if one exists) is structured.

When the *FDA* inspection team requests documents or records, make sure that you record the request and forward it to whoever at your clinic can complete the request (and who you have prepared to assume this role). It is best if you have pre-determined a separate (second) room where document and record requests can be compiled/reviewed prior to submission to the inspectors – rather than in the same room where you are all meeting.

> **Not only should you make sure to keep copies of every document provided to the *FDA* inspectors, but each document and/or record should be watermarked (or stamped) as "confidential."**

(This legally-restricts with whom these *FDA* inspectors can share these documents.)

No matter who you designated to compile/review these documents, it is important that you see them – and hand them to the inspectors yourself. After all, you (assuming you are the legal business owner of your clinic) are the legally responsible person in the eyes of the *FDA* regulators.

If there is an issue in complying with the inspectors' requests for specific documents or records (such as their nonexistence or incomplete state), the person compiling/reviewing these documents or records needs to know that you need to be alerted *privately* – and not verbally in front of the investigators (per your protocol that you developed as part of the project management plan for regulatory inspections). This can be accomplished by texting you, or briefly excusing yourself to talk to the employee you designated as your compiler/reviewer. However, communicating with that person in silence and without leaving the room is far more preferable.

Next, your scribe should make note of any records brought into the room in which you are meeting with the *FDA* inspectors, along with a note of whether they intend to take the documents (which are copies) with them or just review them during the inspection. The inspectors may (or may not) want a tour of your facility at this point.

During any inspection tour, your employee designated for this role and scribe (as well as you) should always accompany them. This can enable you to maintain "control" of the inspection process as much as possible. The last thing you want at this point is a lower-level or dissatisfied employee telling the inspectors something that could lead them to become suspicious of your USP 797 compliance.

As per your SOP for any meetings with *FDA* inspectors, your designated scribe should record what is being reviewed by the inspectors during the tour and any employees/patients being interviewed. If the inspectors request to take photos or videos during the tour, ensure that you know what is essentially encompassed in these photos/videos. If possible, it is a good idea to take photos/videos at the same time for your records.

Notably – if the *FDA* inspectors request to enter clean rooms or other controlled environments – always provide them with the training (per your protocols) necessary to prevent microbiological contamination, and inclusive of donning the proper PPE and following sterile procedure requirements and techniques. Not doing this will suggest to the *FDA* inspectors that you are lax about who can enter your clean rooms and/or following infection control and safety protocols. That is the last impression you want to give to these compliance investigators on the tour of your facility.

As specified in a downloadable document of *Quality Systems Compliance, LLC* available online (from which some of the ideas in this subsection pertaining to step-by-step likely occurrences were abstracted), the *FDA* inspectors are not required to sign your organizational documents, such as:

1. Waivers exempting your clinic from any responsibility (or liability) should an accident occur.
2. Form letters concerning access to confidential information your clinic does not want released.
3. Training forms acknowledging training on personnel PPE (*e.g.*, gowning) procedures.
4. Information/data requests. (The only document that *FDA* inspectors are authorized to sign are "sign-in" and "sign-out

forms" – paper and/or electronic – to comply with security measures.)

MIDDLE STAGE OF THE INSPECTION VISIT

This is where your pre-planning and employee "drills" will really need to have occurred. Do not underestimate what the *FDA* investigators notice as they visit various areas in your clinic! As emphasized earlier in this book, they are looking for evidence of noncompliance with USP 797. Most likely – in addition to wanting to investigate your storage mechanisms (including refrigerator/freezer and the actual supplies that you use in providing IV vitamin perfusions, along with your clean room, patient treatment areas, and even the basement to ascertain any vermin infestations) – they will want to see demonstrations by your clinical staff of how various processes/procedures occur at your health center.

Additionally, *FDA* investigators are likely to want to speak with different employees to corroborate what some other employee has said to them (and especially about adherence to safety and infection control practices). Never underestimate their attentiveness to detail, as these are trained professionals at what they do.

The *American Society of Health-System Pharmacists (ASHP)* suggests that your clinic employees who are involved in providing IV infusions be prepared to answer such questions as the following:

1. Is the air in the negative pressure room vented to the outside?
2. What is the ISO classification of each room in the Clean Room Complex?
3. Are your gowns and gloves sterile or non-sterile?
4. How often do you change your sterile gloves?
5. How often are the isolator hoods cleaned? What agents are used to clean the hoods? What is the spectrum of effectiveness of the cleaning agents? Who inspects the pre-filters in the hoods? How often?

6. How often do you sanitize the bins that go into the clean room?

7. How often do you do surface sampling? How do you pick the sites?

8. What is your cleaning procedure for the hood? What products are you using?

9. Are you using dedicated scrubs and shoes? Describe the gowning procedure.

10. Are you filtering add pools with a 0.22 micron filter? Where are compounds labeled? Describe the final check of compounded product.

11. Who does your hood/room certification? Are they *Controlled Environment Testing Association* (*CETA*)-certified? How do you monitor temperatures and humidity? What is your emergency plan if your HVAC system fails? What is your emergency plan if your refrigerator fails? What is your emergency plan if your electrical power fails? If you have a generator, how do you test it?

12. How are media fill tests conducted? Do you have a control for the media fill tests?

13. Where are your policies and procedures? Who has access to the policies and procedures?

14. Where are your compounding records? What products are compounded in syringes?

15. Have you had any positive [bacterial] results from environmental monitoring? Was it air or surface sampling? How was this handled? Do you perform end-product sampling? Have you had any positive [bacterial] samples? How was this handled?

Your designated employee(s) may also be asked about the compounding pharmacy that supplies you with vitamins, minerals, and other nutrients for provision to patients. Ditto for the vendor supplying saline solutions, gloves/gowns, IV apparatus, and cleaning/disinfection supplies. If that vendor is recognized by investigators as linked to marketing expired, defective, and/or products not allowed to be sold in the US, your safety/infection control compliance will be doubted. As previously mentioned in an earlier chapter, you may be found deficient by the *FDA* investigators for a fault of your *vendor* rather than your clinic or staff.

While this sounds unfair, the investigators consider it your responsibility not to purchase items from such vendors (and especially if the investigators ascertain that some type of supply is defective, such as certain hand-sanitizers containing methanol [wood] alcohol that are no longer allowed to be sold in the US).

As you now truly understand, SOPs and documentation are critical to demonstrating your capacity (and likelihood) of USP 797 compliance. If you were sloppy about creating SOPs and/or documentation, you are most likely going to be caught flat-footed – and need to ensure (and demonstrate) compliance after they generate a report finding you deficient in this area.

LATER STAGE OF THE INSPECTION VISIT AND FINAL THOUGHTS FOR YOUR CONSIDERATION

It is vital for you to be aware that – at any time during the *FDA* investigators' visit to your clinic– these investigators can continue to request specific documentation from you. Throughout the entire inspection, it is important that you always be truthful in whatever you say to them – as lying will most likely be uncovered through their diligent processes, and result in everything else you ever said to them being considered probably "untrue" and "suspect."

Due to the tremendous growth across the US of ambulatory IV infusion centers and the use of IV vitamin infusions by people who are not medically considered in need of these, the *FDA* is scrutinizing them far more than ever before. While a report of an adverse event was the customary past reason prompting an *FDA* 797 compliance visit to a health clinic or business, this situation is changing. One of the primary reasons for this change is that an increasing number of clinics and other businesses are not ensuring that their staff are licensed and/or trained to provide IV vitamin infusions; are poorly managed with sloppy infection control practices; or have deficiencies in terms of site safety (such as malfunctioning patient chairs in the treatment room).

Please do not add to the problem of increased *FDA* inspections by being a clinic that is placing the health of your patients and/or employees at risk. Meanwhile, *do* expect that – at some point in time – that your clinic or wellness center will probably be visited by *FDA* inspectors.

KEY TAKEAWAYS FROM THIS CHAPTER

- Due to the tremendous growth across the US of ambulatory IV infusion centers and the use of IV vitamin infusions by people who are not medically considered in need of these, the *FDA* is scrutinizing centers that provide IV vitamin infusions far more than ever before for compliance with USP 797.
- If your health clinic or other health-related business mixes vitamins into a solution and places this mixture into an intravenous (IV) apparatus for the purpose of infusion into a person, the *FDA* considers this from a regulatory-standpoint as pharmaceutical *manufacturing*.
- If you do not agree with a determination of noncompliance with USP 797 by the *FDA*, you are allowed legally to contact the *FDA*'s Office of the Ombudsman to seek a resolution.

9

WHEN THE DEPARTMENT OF PHARMACY INSPECTS YOUR BUSINESS: WHAT TO EXPECT

T he practice of pharmacy is highly regulated by state laws, and all pharmacies are subject to state Board of Pharmacy inspections. You may not consider your business to be a pharmacy, but you now grasp that – merely by offering IV vitamin infusions – your health clinic or center is considered by pharmacy boards to fall within this classification. For this reason, the first issue that you need to ensure prior to providing any IV vitamin infusion is that your business has a current (and active) pharmacy license, as not having one can result in a dire outcome for your business.

> **News flash. The consequence for your clinic or center to deficiencies in compliance noted upon inspection can be suspension or revocation of that pharmacy license.**

(Please note that any resultant disciplinary action may result in insurance payor/Pharmacy Benefit Manager [PBM] contract terminations, which may – or may not – be applicable to your group practice or center but is important to recognize).

Typically, you can expect that an inspector from a Board of Pharmacy will do the following: 1)identify himself/herself upon arrival with a

Board-issued badge, and provide a business card with all contact information; 2) be professional and courteous throughout the inspection; 3)provide a receipt for any records taken into possession in the course of the inspection; 4)review and leave a copy of the inspection report with you; and 5)provide information and answer questions about pharmacy laws and regulations.[xv]

WHAT IS THE "RIGHT TO INSPECT" AND HOW DOES IT AFFECT THE INSPECTION PROCESS?

Departments of Pharmacy (or Boards of Pharmacy) are legally-granted through *Acts* passed by state legislatures certain authoritative powers. One is the "right to inspect," and this allows state Department (or Board) of Pharmacy inspections to ensure that pharmacies within a given state – *at any time* – meet minimum state and federal standards of operation and practice. As already suggested in the earlier chapter focused on preparing for contact by a regulatory authority, Boards of Pharmacy routinely inspect pharmacies for diverse reasons, including the following: inspections prior to permitting/licensing; inspections after receipt of an application for change of location or change of ownership; routine periodic inspections to ensure compliance; and enforcement inspections.

It is the category of "enforcement inspections" that is enabling Boards of Pharmacy to assign inspectors to undertake inspections of IV infusion centers whenever they choose to conduct that inspection – and regardless of whether they provide advance notification to you or not.

Historically, routine inspections have occurred to assess compliance with state statutes and regulations. In contrast, enforcement inspections were normally triggered by a complaint or threat of danger to the public (or as a follow-up to ensure corrective actions were implemented after prior violations had been identified by inspectors). However, this has changed due to the high number of reported injuries resulting from infections resultant from compounded pharmaceuticals (such as provided in IV infusion centers). Therefore, a key takeaway from this section is to understand that a pharmacy (or health center deemed as one) should not refuse an inspection, as such a refusal is generally considered an independent violation of state pharmacy regulatory law.

CHECKLISTS AND FORMS THAT MAY BE APPLICABLE TO YOUR BUSINESS

There are many checklists/forms utilized by the state Board of Pharmacy in determining whether the inspected pharmacy is in compliance – or is *not* compliant. By familiarizing yourself with these, you may be able to take specific advance actions to increase the likelihood of your business being determined as compliant by the inspectors that visit your clinic or wellness center to inspect it. The inspector(s) that visit your clinic or wellness center typically bring specific checklists or forms that are completed by these regulatory employees on the day of the inspection. Generally-speaking, these checklists/forms fall into the following two different categories: 1) those applying to retail and hospital outpatient facilities, and 2) those applying to compounding pharmacies (such as your IV vitamin infusion center).

In order for you to be able to understand the commonalities and differences between the checklists within these two categories (along with gleaning the types of issues that you need to address well in advance of an inspection), both categories are described below.

ITEMS COMMONLY INCLUDED IN THE CHECKLIST/FORMS OF RETAIL AND HOSPITAL OUTPATIENT PHARMACIES:

1. Original pharmacy license and current renewal displayed.
2. Current US *Drug Enforcement Administration (DEA)* registration.
3. Pharmacist and pharmacy technician nametags, current licensure, and required annual Continuing Education Unit (CEU) completion.
4. Pharmacist-in-charge duties.

5. Pharmacist duties (other than for Pharmacist-in-Charge).
6. Pharmacy technician duties.
7. Advanced practice pharmacist duties.
8. Facility has adequate security (including an alarmed security system and working security cameras; heating and air conditioning available and working; and posted business hours).
9. Security and storage of pharmacy area, medications, and records.
10. Appropriate and clean pharmacy department workspace (including the size of an area, adequate lighting, access to sinks with hot and cold water, temperature of the refrigeration system, and readily accessible bathroom).
11. Appropriate equipment (*e.g.*, counting devices, devices capable of measuring volumes) necessary to dispense, label, and distribute drugs.
12. Appropriate reference books and state Board of Pharmacy rules.
13. Suitable patient consultation area.
14. Proper supervision of pharmacy staff.
15. Drug stock is clean, orderly, properly-stored, and properly-labeled.
16. Drugs are purchased from a licensed wholesaler or manufacturer.
17. Receipt/distribution of drugs.
18. Prescription requirements compliance.
19. Prescription labeling, furnishing, dispensing, and storage.
20. Prescription transfers.
21. Prescription confidentiality.
22. Refill authorization and documentation.
23. Drug utilization review.
24. Prescription Monitoring Program (PMP) compliance.
25. Documented quality assurance/quality improvement and medication errors identification/review program.
26. Books and recordkeeping (includes prescription dispensing, prescription transfers, patient profiles, purchase invoices and

receipts, controlled substances, inventory records, logbook records, returns, and destroyed drugs).

27. Appropriate records storage.
28. Appropriate *DEA* forms and controlled substances inventory records.
29. Corresponding responsibility for controlled substances prescriptions.
30. Policies and procedures.
31. Automated dispensing devices.
32. Re-packaging/pre-packaging.
33. Outdated, damaged, and recalled drugs are segregated.

ITEMS COMMONLY INCLUDED IN THE CHECKLIST/FORMS OF COMPOUNDING PHARMACIES:

1. Compounding limitations and requirements (preparation timing, storage, office use, *FDA*-prohibited, master formula, bulk chemicals, Beyond Use Dates [BUDs], and stability studies).
2. Recordkeeping (master formula; compound certificate of analysis, compounding log accurately maintained; acquisition, storage, and destruction of chemicals, active chemical acquisitions, and dispensing records).
3. Labeling requirements (active/therapeutic ingredients).
4. Compounding policies and procedures.
5. Compounding facilities and equipment functioning and maintained (testing and calibration; cleaning and disinfecting; hood certification).
6. Training of compounding staff (such as documentation of aseptic training).
7. Compounding quality assurance (such as adverse effects/complaints documented and investigated, and recalls and prescriber/patient notifications conducted when required).
8. Compounding for parenteral therapy.
9. Sterile compounding from non-sterile ingredients.

10. Sterile compounding area.
11. Sterile compounding attire.
12. Sterile compounding quality assurance and process validation.
13. Beyond Use Dating (BUD) for sterile compounded drug preparations.
14. Limitations on use of single-dose and multi-dose containers.
15. Compounding reference materials.
16. Sterile compounding certification/licensure.

SOME THINGS TO REMEMBER DURING THE INSPECTION – WHAT YOU CAN DO

As cited in an article in the *Journal of Health Care Compliance* for many points discussed in this chapter, the following are some things for you to remember or do during the actual inspection:

1. Require the Board of Pharmacy inspector(s) to show their State Board of Pharmacy credentials upon arrival. (Due to the increasing prevalence of people attempting to "scam" small businesses and individuals, it is more important than ever before to ensure that the people arriving at your business are indeed Board of Pharmacy inspectors – and not imposters posing as inspectors.)
2. Ask questions about the audit's scope and goals, and record the answers given for pharmacy records.
3. Establish a designated room or area where the Board of Pharmacy inspector(s) may meet with staff, review documents, or ask their questions.
4. Require staff to be polite and respectful to the inspector and truthfully respond to questions asked (albeit without offering more information than required and/or necessary).
5. Instruct staff not to speculate (or guess) if unsure of a response to a question. Additionally – if the question is unclear – your staff member should ask that it be re-phrased.
6. Prohibit staff members from admitting to any violations of

law (either federal or state) or regulations. If they believe there is a violation of some type – rather than state it – they should just request that the instructors talk to you (or your specific designee) directly.

7. Instruct staff to respond only to questions asked, and not to offer or otherwise volunteer information in addition to that necessary to respond to the question.

8. Require your designated employee to take notes during the inspection process, including (but not limited to) questions asked, statements made, documents requested and reviewed, comments made by the Board of Pharmacy inspector(s), and responses to them.

9. Do not permit the inspector unsupervised, free access to records, documents, or files unless legally entitled to that access (with proof shown beforehand of that legal entitlement).

10. Provide copies of any requested documents.

11. Keep the originals and document any records provided (*i.e.,* document with the date/time and recipient of the records for your own record-keeping).

12. Conduct an exit meeting to determine any issues identified in the inspection audit and ask for the list of any discrepancies in writing.

13. The pharmacy/pharmacist/manager should not sign any documents that acknowledge any specific findings or commit to any corrective actions prior to consulting with your lawyer or legal team.

POST-INSPECTION FOLLOW-UP – KEY POINTS FOR YOU TO REMEMBER

1. The pharmacy/pharmacist/manager should share and discuss the results of the Board of Pharmacy inspection with your lawyers (if these were not present) – and then should immediately formulate responses to identified deficiencies, including consideration of policy and procedure, facility, or

equipment changes that could address the issues raised by the inspector(s).

2. Investigate any potential problems that arose during the Board of Pharmacy inspection audit. Consult with your lawyers to clarify issues and concerns.

3. All Board of Pharmacy inspector requests for follow-up submission of additional documents or responses to specific questions should be answered as soon as reasonably possible.

4. Once the written inspection report detailing the full audit findings is complete, review it carefully to make sure it matches the notes taken during the inspection.

5. Work with your lawyers to prepare and forward a rebuttal response before the specified deadline with copies of any supporting documentation needed.

6. If disciplinary action is taken, then consult with your lawyers regarding an administrative hearing or appeal.

Do not forget that the inspector is allowed to take samples of compounded products (such as vitamin solutions that are IV-administered at your health clinic), so – if there is some problem found with that compounded product – you may receive notification of the problem *after* the inspector has left your premises. An analysis by a state government employee who is a chemist may need to occur, which can take additional time for a compliance determination to be issued. My point is that – while you may have some sense of whether the inspector is going to find your health clinic deficient in some compliance aspect following departure – this is definitely not always the case.

As previously recommended in preparing for any type of regulatory inspection, it is a good idea to designate a particular employee as your "point person" for dealing with the entire inspection process. Remember: this involves your identifying one suitable employee to field questions from the inspector. In this way, you can minimize the disruption at your health clinic or center, as well as ensure that the responses are consistent with internal policies and procedures/SOPs focused on "actions" at your clinic during inspections. Of course, any key employee that you designate must be knowledgeable as to the limitations on the breadth and scope of inspection authority, and also be familiar with all of your relevant policies and procedures.

ACTIONS THAT CAN OCCUR AS A RESULT OF AN INSPECTOR DETERMINATION OF DEFICIENCIES IN COMPLIANCE

If the Board of Pharmacy inspector suspects that your business is not in compliance, you will most likely receive a written notice of that determination (if your business is not immediately closed by the inspector due to deficiencies discovered during the inspection). Depending on the type of violation as determined by the Board of Pharmacy, there are – at minimum – three standard Board of Pharmacy legal actions that occur. These are: 1)issuance of a letter of admonishment; 2) issuance of a citation (with or without a fine of monies); and 3) referral of the case for disciplinary action against the business and/or you as the business owner.

A Letter of Admonishment will most likely detail the deficiencies identified by the inspection and allow you to respond. That response can be either one that argues against the deficiency or demonstrates how (and when) you can correct the deficiency. If you receive a Letter of Admonishment (or other letter similar in content), your health clinic or center may be either prevented from providing IV infusions or temporarily closed during the time period that you are correcting the identified deficiencies in compliance.

Meanwhile, if you also receive a citation requiring payment of a fine to the state, your health clinic or center may be temporary closed not only until the deficiencies are corrected but until the fined amount is paid with documentation of receipt. Disciplinary action that goes beyond a fine against your business, your Medical Director, (or you) is the most severe Board of Pharmacy inspection consequence, and it is likely to result in the involvement of other governmental regulatory entities as well as closure of your health clinic or center for a longer period of time or permanently.

Whatever you do in terms of responding to a Board of Pharmacy written communication of compliance deficiencies identified during an inspection, you will probably need qualified and knowledgeable legal counsel to help you to formulate your response in a way that will not make things worse for you. On the other hand, many IV infusion centers do not have compliance deficiencies identified because they prepared themselves as recommended in this book – so you may not encounter any negative consequences from a Board of Pharmacy inspection.

KEY TAKEAWAYS FROM THIS CHAPTER

- Boards of Pharmacy (or Departments of Pharmacy) are legally-granted through *Acts* passed by state legislatures such authoritative powers as the "right to inspect." This allows inspections by state Boards of Pharmacy to ensure that pharmacies within a state *at any time* meet minimum state and federal standards of operation and practice.
- It is a good idea in engaging in the steps to prepare your health center for an inspection to designate one particular employee as the "point person" to field questions from the inspector and to oversee the entire inspection.
- There are many checklists/forms utilized by a state Board of Pharmacy in determining whether the inspected pharmacy is in regulatory compliance. By familiarizing yourself with these checklists/forms, you may be able to take specific advance actions to increase the likelihood of your health center receiving a determination of compliance upon a Board of Pharmacy inspection.

10

WHEN YOUR STATE BOARD OF HEALTH INSPECTS YOUR BUSINESS: WHAT TO EXPECT

E very state in the US has a Department of Public Health (DPH) or some agency charged with a similar public health role. While nearly all DPHs have regulatory authority related to the licensure of outpatient health clinics, only a small number of states have granted their DPHs licensing authority not only of health clinics but specifically of med spas and naturopathic centers offering IV vitamin infusions. If your business is located in a state where you are required to have a DPH-provided license (such as Massachusetts), you have to meet DPH regulatory requirements as well as those of your Department of Pharmacy (along with other state and local regulatory entities).

Not only has nationwide awareness of adverse events at compounding pharmacies and outpatient IV infusion centers increased, but the onset of the Covid-19 pandemic has increased nationwide awareness of the infection prevention roles of state Departments of Public Health. Indeed, the Covid-19 pandemic has promoted far greater oversight of health centers (inclusive of outpatient IV infusion centers) than ever before. One of the major reasons is that so many people who receive outpatient IV infusions of prescription medications and/or vitamins have lowered immune systems – with their immunocompromised health status placing them at higher risk of acquiring a severe Covid-19 infection.

But, it is also important to understand the impact of the Corporate Practice of Medicine (CPOM) doctrine on DPH-generated regulations governing licensure.

OVERALL IMPACT OF CORPORATE PRACTICE OF MEDICINE (CPOM) DOCTRINE

The corporate practice of medicine (CPOM) doctrine prohibits corporations from practicing medicine or employing a physician to provide professional medical services. This doctrine arose from state medical practice legislative *Acts*. As described by the *American Medical Association (AMA)*, CPOM doctrine was based on a number of public policy concerns. These included the following widely-held medical practitioner beliefs: 1)allowing corporations to practice medicine or employ physicians will result in the commercialization of the practice of medicine; 2) a corporation's obligation to its shareholders may not align with a physician's obligation to his patients; and 3) employment of a physician by a corporation may interfere with the physician's independent medical judgment.

It is vital to realize that most states have regulations prohibitive of – to greater or lesser extent – the corporate practice of medicine. On the other hand, most states have broad exceptions (such as for *Accountable Care Organizations* [*ACOs*] and employment of physicians by certain healthcare-related entities). Meanwhile, some states do allow non-physician owners or shareholders. The reason this matters is that – depending upon your state's CPOM laws – ownership of a wellness center or med spa (regardless of whether IV vitamin infusions are offered) can result in license revocation and/or the inability to obtain a license for your health clinic from the DPH.

REPORTS AND COMPLAINTS TO THE DEPARTMENT OF PUBLIC HEALTH – IMPLICATIONS FOR YOUR CLINIC

The DPH is most likely to require an inspection prior to obtaining your license to operate as an outpatient health clinic or due to a report of an adverse event. If the inspection occurs as the result of an adverse event (such as an infection in one of your patients/clients caused by an unsterile needle inserted to provide the IV vitamin infusion) or complaints about your facility, the inspection can result in the closure of your health clinic.

State DPHs provide information on state residents' infections to the US *Centers for Disease Control* (*CDC*), so a cluster of Covid-19 cases linked to your health clinic could result in federal regulatory inspections and permanently-increased scrutiny by regulatory authorities.

DEPARTMENTS OF PUBLIC HEALTH AND COMPOUNDING PHARMACIES – DETERMINATION OF CONTAMINANTS

One of the roles of most DPHs is to analyze substances suspected of causing medical crises and infections. Collaboratively, they are often the governmental entities that determine if a diagnosed infection was caused by a specific medication or vitamin infusion. The testimony of DPH chemists can be used in a court of law, and inspection by the DPH of your health clinic is likely if a compounding pharmacy that provides vitamin packages to you (such as *Myers' Cocktail* packages containing a mix of magnesium, calcium, B-vitamins, andvitaminC) is cited for any reason – but especially for contaminated products. For this reason, it bears repeating that you really do need to be aware of any legal citations against your vendors. Otherwise, you could become ensnared in a DPH action against that vendor.

DEPARTMENTS OF PUBLIC HEALTH AND COVID-19 INFECTION CONTROL POLICIES

Consequent to the Covid-19 pandemic, state regulations have empowered DPHs to enforce increased respiratory infection control measures in indoor facilities (such as health clinics and wellness centers). These measures include but are not limited to: 1) daily Covid-19 testing of all outpatient healthcare clinic employees (and non-allowance of anyone testing positive to enter the clinic); 2) face-mask wearing by all patients/clients and employees; 3) specific maximum number of people allowed in the outpatient clinic at any one time; 4) specific social distancing requirements (such as maintaining six feet of distance between each patient/client); 5)specific cleaning and disinfection protocols aimed at preventing Covid-19 spread; 6) vaccination against Covid-19 by all clinicians; and 7) disallowance of anyone (whether employee or patient) to remain in the clinic if exhibiting an increased body temperature plus other symptoms suggestive of Covid-19 infection.

Presently, there are an increasing number of localities within states that are requiring proof of Covid-19 vaccination by anyone entering a healthcare clinic or wellness center.

Violations of state and local health regulations and policies resulting from the ongoing Covid-19 pandemic can also result in revocation of site license, citation (with or without financial penalty), and/or closure of your clinic or business. Therefore, it is extremely important that you keep "current" on all Covid-19 infection control regulations and take them seriously. Failure to adhere can not only jeopardize the health of your employees and patients/clients, but it can result in an unwanted DPH regulatory reaction while also ruining your clinic's overall reputation. You can be sure that – if there is an outbreak of Covid-19 at your clinic, that news will travel around your community quickly.

KEY TAKEAWAYS FROM THIS CHAPTER

- If your health center providing IV infusions is located in a state where you are required to have a license granted by the state Department of Public Health (DPH), you have to meet state DPH regulatory requirements as well as those of the Department of Pharmacy. For this reason, you need to familiarize yourself with the laws of your state pertaining to IV infusion centers.

- The Corporate Practice of Medicine (CPOM) doctrine prohibits corporations from practicing medicine or employing a physician to provide professional medical services. Depending upon your state's CPOM laws, corporate ownership of a health center or med spa (regardless of whether IV vitamin infusions are offered) may result in license revocation and/or the inability to obtain a DPH-issued license for your health-related business.
- If there is an infection outbreak or adverse health event at your health center or health-related business, the Department of Public Health (DPH) of your state is likely to become involved as well as the Department of Pharmacy of your state and the US *Food and Drug Administration (FDA)*.

11

EVALUATION OF YOUR EMPLOYEE TRAININGS AND INCORPORATING USEFUL STAFF FEEDBACK

I t is not enough to provide training (and re-training) to your clinicians and other staff of your health clinic or wellness center that is providing IV vitamin infusions. You need to be able to evaluate both whether your employees have learned something from their attendance in a given training session *and* whether they utilize what they have learned in order to foster USP 797 compliance.

For example, a specific training session for a clinician who performs IV vitamin infusions might be focused on the *Infusion Nurses' Society (INS)* vitamin infusion standards in relation to osmolality (the concentration of a solution expressed as the total number of solute particles per kilogram [kg]). Meanwhile, a specific training session for medical assistants supporting clinicians who perform IV vitamin infusions might be focused on acquiring, documenting, and reporting vital signs (*e.g.,* blood pressure) of a patient/client prior to placement of an IV for a vitamin infusion. For any training series (inclusive of each individual session), clear learning objectives needed to be presented at the beginning of the session and provided as a hand-out to the employees as "students."

Meanwhile, the trainers for the training programs (including each training session in the training program) need to be knowledgeable in the subject matter and excellent instructors. Therefore, it is not going to be sufficient to have existing employees conducting the training sessions for attendance by other employees. Instead, you are going to have to hire qualified and skilled trainers who are up-to-date on "best practices" in the corresponding subject matter and the teaching of it.

However, compliance alone does not demonstrate whether your employees understood what they learned in a training program (and/or its individual sessions). You will also need to have someone construct a framework for evaluating your employees in their on-the-job performance of what was taught in the sessions. While you may have a management employee competent enough to construct that framework, more likely you will need to pay an outside contractor skilled in training and evaluation methods to do this for you.

The element of surprise is important in gauging whether a given employee is utilizing what they learned in the training session. One major reason the element of surprise is so important is that Department of Pharmacy, Department of Public Health, and *FDA* inspectors are going to surprise you and your employees when they show up at your health clinic. Therefore, engaging the element of surprise is important for evaluating whether your employees are acting on a daily basis in compliance with USP 797 regulations and "best practices."

Likewise, obtaining feedback following training sessions from your employees is an important component of evaluation. Since an employee may be reluctant to provide honest feedback (due to a perception that such feedback could impact their performance evaluation from a personnel standpoint or impact other employees), the mechanism for obtaining feedback needs to ensure that the employee cannot be identified. Moreover, the individual responses prior to session feedback response analysis need to be kept confidential from all other employees and you. Only in this way will your employees feel free to provide negative feedback that is not constrained by fear of retaliation.

Of course, any feedback that provides useful information – such as a majority of attendees of a particular training session responding that the material covered was outdated – needs to be used to adjust the training (and the instructor of that training) accordingly.

IN-PERSON OR ONLINE TRAINING, TESTING, AND EVALUATION – WHICH IS BETTER?

You may feel that online training is more productive than having your employees (especially your non-clinical employees) attend training sessions on work time. Ditto for reading training books and taking a test. Whichever route you choose, it should be the one that is most effective at enabling your employees to learn the required information. Moreover – since USP 797 requires that a compound pharmacy perform employee training and re-training – documenting everything pertaining to each training program/session is imperative (inclusive of PowerPoint slides and/or hand-outs used/provided in each session).

One of the key things to remember when any written tests are utilized as part of an evaluation mechanism following a training is that "cheating" has to be prevented. In other words – if employees take a test in a training room – there needs to be enough distance between employees so that they cannot read the answers on a test provided by another employee as "student." If the test is offered online, it can be even more difficult to ensure that someone else does not take the test *in place of* the employee enrolled in the training session in an effort to "cheat." (While the trend is for online training and testing, it can be more difficult to control cheating with the use of this training mode.)

Utilizing online evaluation software can be a good way to conduct training evaluations, but there will need to be a way to ensure that a given employee is not compromised if an email address is required by the software to begin the online evaluation. Otherwise, the honesty of the employee's evaluation responses may be compromised due to a lack of full anonymity.

I cannot emphasize enough that training is a continuous and ongoing process in order for it to make a difference in terms of keeping your health clinic center in regulatory compliance. Yes, it will cost you in terms of time and money, but it will be worth it if it enables you not to be found deficient in USP 797 compliance.

This chapter is intentionally short because training normally requires your delegation to competent trainers to carry out the necessary training, testing, and evaluation. My final point is to remind you to enable your top-level management employee overseeing training programs at your health center to adjust the trainings in response to useful employee feedback. Just because a specific approach worked in the past does not mean it is the best approach now. You will need to be flexible enough to adjust to new training "best practices" when it comes to training your employees whether clinical or nonclinical.

KEY TAKEAWAYS FROM THIS CHAPTER

- You need to be able to evaluate both whether the employees at your health center or other health-related business have learned something from their attendance in any given training session, as well as whether they utilize what they have learned in order to boost USP 797 compliance.
- In order to ensure that employee training sessions increases knowledge level and skill capacity to achieve and maintain USP 797 compliance, you are going to have to hire qualified and skilled trainers who are up-to-date on "best practices" in the corresponding subject matter *and* the teaching of that subject matter. This includes the capacity of trainers to evaluate the effectiveness of the training sessions.
- Training and evaluation need to be performed on an ongoing basis in order for these to make an obvious difference in terms of keeping your health clinic center in regulatory compliance. While the investment in employee training/re-training may initially seem not to be worth the financial cost to you, it will clearly be worthwhile it if it reduces the likelihood of inspectors concluding your noncompliance with USP 797.

12

EVALUATIONS CONDUCTED INTERNALLY AND YOUR USP 797 COMPLIANCE

Evaluations are essential for you to know if you really are prepared for inspectors from a Board of Pharmacy or other regulatory entity to conduct a USP 797 compliance inspection of your health center or clinic. Following the development and implementation of your project management plan for USP 797 compliance, the best way to ensure that you are prepared for that regulatory inspection is by conducting periodic evaluations/audits.

Below are some of the clustered questions you need to answer through the conduction of evaluations at your health clinic or center.

1. Does the documentation needed to show evidence of USP 797 compliance to regulatory inspectors exist? If so, is that documentation complete (*i.e.,* include a date/time and initials of documenter)? Is the documentation accurate? Can the designated staff easily access the documentation to ascertain what has been done or not yet done, and document whatever they are required to document? Can you easily access the documentation to show it to inspectors upon request?

2. Are infection control measures being carried out according to your SOPs? Are safety measures aimed at patients/clients, employees, and visitors being carried out according to internal policies?

3. Are your employees performing only the roles actually assigned to them (*e.g.,* only clinicians performing roles involving clinical functions per their licensed clinician status)? Do you have adequate staffing in any and all roles needed to provide IV vitamin infusions under USP 797? Are your clinical staff licensed to perform their roles, and are their licenses current/active?

4. Are all of your employees "up-to-date" in their training and employment role-based "best practices" knowledge? Are trainings being conducted regularly, and are evaluations of each training session occurring (inclusive of obtaining employees' feedback as students)?

5. Is your building and all facilities in compliance with all state and federal laws? Are all required facility-related infection control and safety measures in place (such as an adequate ventilation system and unblocked building/room exists in case of emergency)?

6. Is everything utilized to provide care to patients/clients in proper working order, properly cleaned and disinfected, and available when needed? Have any potential health hazards (such as inadequate airing out of rooms following floor-washing with ammonia-based products) not been prevented or corrected? Are licenses for elevators (if such exist) current/active?

7. Is every piece of equipment and item/substance utilized for the compounding of anything for use in IV vitamin administration documented with the name and contact information of the vendor/supplier, date last serviced (if equipment), expiration date, and anything else required for USP 797 compliance as well as infection control/safety? Are refrigerators and heating systems always maintained at the correct temperature and in proper working order? Do designated employees conduct regularly-scheduled "checks" for recalls, Beyond Use Dates (BUDs), and everything else required for UPS 797 compliance as per the health center's SOPs? Is sterile compounding procedure always followed?

8. Is the disposal of everything utilized in your health center occurring as specified in your SOPs for infection control and safety? Are any

mistakes or problems related to disposal identified quickly and documented?

9. Do all employees understand to whom they report any errors linked to infection control, safety, and/or USP 797 compliance? Are they following SOPs in this arena? If not, why not? Are all adverse events experienced by patients/clients, employees, or visitors (including external vendors and repair-persons) of any kind at the clinic being reported, documented, and addressed?

10. Are your employees prepared for a USP 797 regulatory inspection by a federal or state regulatory entity? How can you better prepare your employees (and facility) for an unplanned (surprise) visit by inspectors?

These are just some of the many questions that you need to answer for yourself through implementation of an internal evaluation mechanism. In other words, one of the projects within your project management framework needs to be "in-house" evaluations and audits that can continuously supply the answers to questions such as these to you at any given time.

PROJECT MANAGEMENT SOFTWARE AND CREATING A PROJECT MANAGEMENT PLAN FOR EVALUATIONS

You may already have guessed that you will likely need to utilize project management software to stay "on top" of all of the components of your action planning pertaining to evaluations. If you have more than two employees, you will probably need project management software rather than simply using a spreadsheet or "pen and paper." There are many different types available for purchase, or you may prefer to have an Information Technology (IT) firm that designs project management software specifically aimed at clients' needs create a proprietary one for you. Whichever route you choose to acquire project management software, you (and your designated employees) will need to learn how to utilize that software.

INTERNAL EVALUATION PROCESS TO ASSESS REGULATORY RISK

A *Journal of Business Compliance* article was focused on "best practices" for the management of regulatory risk within project management, and included a description of common shortfalls in regulatory compliance preparedness in project planning (as well as suggested measures to assist project managers in planning for – and meeting – regulatory requirements). This article's descriptions are the source of most of what is presented in this subsection of this chapter. Meanwhile, one conclusion expressed in this article is: "Experience shows that compliance should be integrated into a project at its conception and needs to be followed up until the project is completed."

UNDERSTANDING PROJECT MANAGEMENT COMPLIANCE BASICS

The following are presented in the above-noted article as essential elements of project management compliance basics:

1. Include the regulatory impact assessment process as at project initiation.
2. Add compliance to schedule of tasks.
3. Assign regulatory management responsibility.
4. Map and understand regulatory requirements.
5. Know the regulators and their expectations.
6. Establish and maintain a dialog with regulators.
7. Monitor for any changes in regulation.
8. Be aware of regulatory overlap and conflict.
9. Confront compliance difficulties with candor.
10. Respect the internal compliance approval and regulatory appeal processes.

Obviously, you will need to incorporate these project management regulatory compliance basics into your framework for your "in-house" evaluation project management.

HOW CONDUCTING INTERNAL COMPLIANCE EVALUATIONS BUILDS REGULATOR TRUST

One of the lesser-recognized positive impacts of conducting USP 797 compliance evaluations/audits is that it promotes the building of confidence and trust in regulators. In turn, this confidence and trust that you are "on top" of things at your health clinic or center can lead to fewer inspections. In contrast, not demonstrating a project management framework for regulatory compliance – which is basically required under USP 797 – can lead to decreased trust and more frequent inspections. Therefore – despite the resources required to create and maintain an internal evaluation project management (such as time and cost) – it is well worth the effort.

"BEST PRACTICES" FOR MANAGING COMPLIANCE

The 10 "best practices" identified in the aforementioned article are as follows:

1. Start the regulatory process at project initiation.

This article recommends that you need to engage with experts for ensuring regulatory compliance; identify the applicable regulatory agencies with regulatory authority over your business; and dedicate resources to ensure ongoing regulatory compliance.

2. Add compliance to the work schedule.

In other words, you need to build in time (as a project management resource) to manage the projects such as the entire internal evaluation mechanism required for compliance. Likewise, you need to build in time for each project management component (such as clinician training in up-to-date IV vitamin administration).

3. Assign regulatory management responsibility.

There should be a centralized overall manager (such as a designated Compliance Officer). However, the designation of a Compliance Officer does not eliminate the need for the designation of other employees to engage in management of regulatory-related activities. On the other hand, it does mean that there should be one designated employee in the role of Compliance Officer who needs to be informed of all regulatory activities *and* should be charged with the authority to make changes to processes and procedures to ensure compliance.

4. Know the requirements for compliance.

It is imperative that your project managers understand the regulations and are kept abreast of changes to them. Besides reviewing the regulations in their entirety, the project managers (and especially the Compliance Officer) can derive a further understanding by reviewing the most common deficiencies found by a state regulatory entity (such as a Department of Pharmacy) and/or federal regulatory entity (such as the *FDA*) in the past year. In this way, project managers can have a better grasp of areas to which inspectors are likely to pay particular attention. Likewise, project managers need to review any recent safety bulletins and enforcement actions. This can have an added benefit of enabling project managers to appear more competent in the eyes of regulatory inspectors.

5. Know the regulators.

By knowing all regulatory authorities (inclusive of their directors' names and contact information plus usual outcomes of their inspections) that can send an inspector to your health clinic or center, you can be more prepared for an inspection by these regulatory authorities.

6. Establish and maintain a dialog with the regulators.

Consider your relationship with regulators as a collaborative project. In this way, you can engage in more productive interactions as opposed to approaching them with an adversarial mind-set. Something to bear in mind is that your attitude toward regulators will likely translate to your Compliance Officer's attitude toward them, and therefore your employees' attitudes toward them. The negative outcome could be that the inspectors sense this adversarial attitude, so a collaborative attitude can make them more willing to be flexible in their interactions about meeting their compliance standards with you.

7. Monitor for changes in regulation.

This is crucial to meeting regulatory compliance. However, it can also help you to gauge trends for the future in terms of regulations.

8. Be aware of regulatory overlap and conflict.

As discussed in earlier chapters, regulatory authorities that can require compliance to their regulations can be federal, state, and local. Additionally, they may be professional organizations and other licensing entities. It is vital to understand where requirements related to permits or procedures differ between regulatory authorities so that you can find some way to meet the overlapping requirements of each of these authorities.

9. Be upfront with compliance difficulties.

You may find that the time frame allowed in an inspector's report for meeting a specific compliance requirement is totally unrealistic for your health clinic or center. Letting the regulatory authority know your inability to accomplish compliance within the allowed time frame may enable you to acquire more time. The key point herein is to attempt to work collaboratively with regulatory authorities to proactively address a compliance issue, and especially where the requirements of one regulatory authority conflict with that of another. For example, obtaining a local permit to expand your site may take longer than the time you have been allowed to enlarge a compounding room – so enabling your state Department of Pharmacy to understand this may enable them to determine a more realistic time frame for you to renovate your compounding room.

10. Know the legal appeal process.

It is important to recognize that a particular inspector may not have any background in what your health center offers and/or IV vitamin infusions. Likewise, some inspectors are more knowledgeable in terms of recent regulation changes and experienced than others. However, most will realize that you have the legal right to talk to a higher regulatory authority in their agency as needed. It is not the responsibility of the inspector who visits your health clinic to know your legal rights, which is why you need to understand them – and enable your Compliance Officer to understand them.

All the points addressed in this chapter are applicable to the project management of internal evaluations. Yet, there is one other critical point that requires inclusion. This is the need for you to incorporate the following into every aspect of your project management plan for conducting internal evaluations: 1) cost (financial resources needed); 2) time (yours and that of your employees); and 3) resources (material [*e.g.,* binders] and people needed to accomplish that evaluation). Yes, the project management plan needs to be realistic for it to be implemented. Otherwise, it will remain an unrealized action plan, not utilized by anyone, and so not helpful in accomplishing your goal of ensuring USP 797 compliance.

KEY TAKEAWAYS FROM THIS CHAPTER

- Periodic internal evaluations are essential for you to know if you really are prepared for inspectors from a Board of Pharmacy or other regulatory entity to conduct a USP 797 compliance inspection of your health center or other health-related business.
- It is important for you to be aware of regulatory overlap and conflict between various governmental regulatory authorities that may conduct an inspection of your wellness center or other health-related business. This knowledge can enable you to better prepare to address concerns by a particular inspection team regarding your USP 797 compliance.
- One of the lesser-recognized positive impacts of conducting USP 797 compliance evaluations/audits is that it may promote the building of confidence and trust in people in

governmental employment inspection roles that arrive at your health center. In turn, this confidence and trust that you are "on top" of things at your health clinic or center may lead to fewer inspections by that governmental regulatory authority.

13

CONCLUDING THOUGHTS AND IDEAS FOR YOUR NEXT STEPS

You now understand why you need to comply with USP 797 and *how* to comply with it. There has been a huge amount of information condensed into this book in order for you to have a broad understanding of the scope of USP 797 and range of issues that you need to address to adhere to it. Through reading each chapter of this book, you also now comprehend that – simply by providing IV vitamin infusions – your health clinic, wellness center, or other health-related business is considered a compounding pharmacy under the guidelines of the US *Pharmacopeia* (USP) which is enforceable by governmental regulatory authorities.

As a key takeaway from this book, you also comprehend that your health center is considered a *sterile* compounding pharmacy (due to infusions that allow something to enter the recipient's bloodstream). This means that the applicable "best practices" for compounding are even more stringent than otherwise, and resultant from the increased potential for blood infections linked to unsafe practices.

This is essential to remember:

The fact that you must adhere to USP 797 requirements does not mean that your business cannot also be required to adhere to the regulations of other USP chapters, but you are going to be expected to adhere to USP 797 requirements regardless of whether you do any actual combining of vitamins (such as combining Vitamin B12 with Magnesium) or it is done elsewhere.

Let us consider how much you have probably learned from taking the time out of your busy days to read each chapter this book. First of all, you now understand that your provision of IV vitamin infusions means that power has been legally granted by local, state, and federal regulatory entities for regulatory inspections to occur at your center to ascertain compliance with their respective regulations. Likewise, you now know – at the state level – regulatory inspections are usually promulgated by your state's Department of Pharmacy and Department of Public Health. Meanwhile, at the federal level, a regulatory inspection is usually promulgated by the US *Food and Drug Administration (FDA)*.

I cannot emphasize the following point enough for you. Stated bluntly, your health clinic or wellness center is most likely going to be inspected by a governmental regulatory authority if you offer IV infusions of any kind. As you are now well aware, the requirements to meet USP 797 compliance can differ between regulatory authorities – and especially between state and federal regulatory authorities. This can make compliance feel even more confusing for you.

Money, money, money. Now that I have your attention, let us move on to one topic only minimally addressed in this book:

Your business plan's budget section may not have included costs associated with USP 797 – and your monthly revenues may not even cover your monthly expenditures if your health center is new. Yes, the cost of compliance in terms of monies needed to meet USP requirements can be steep (and probably adversely impact your net worth in the short term).

However, the cost of *noncompliance* can be even steeper in terms of the consequences. These consequences include infection or accidental injury that can both damage your business reputation and result in governmental-instituted closure of your business and other legal actions against you. For this reason, you do need to set aside monies to ensure your USP 797 compliance if you plan to offer (or already offer) IV infusions to your patients/clients.

Hopefully, this book has enabled you to feel less powerless in your interactions with state and federal regulators if you have not yet dealt with a regulatory inspection. Likewise, it is also my hope that reading this book has helped you to grasp what you need to do if you have been found upon an inspection to be deficient in some aspect of compliance. Most of all, my fervent hope is that you will utilize this book as a reference for yourself to make your health center as USP 797-compliant as possible, so that regulators will get "out of your hair" due to the high compliance standards you have placed on yourself. After all, the more regulators are satisfied with your compliance, the less likely they will be to make frequent *re-inspection* visits to your clinic.

In summary, the key takeaway of this book is to be proactive in ensuring that an inspector from any regulatory authority will not find your outpatient medical practice, health clinic, or wellness center deficient in USP 797 compliance or consider your provision of IV vitamin infusions to be placing the recipients at a health and/or safety risk. Although regulations enacted for infection control and safety reasons can seem like a major nuisance for health clinics (and health-related businesses), these types of regulations were enacted to protect people's health and safety. Therefore, ensuring that your health clinic is following "best practices" per USP 797 demonstrates that you take public health and safety seriously.

My educational program and templates can be found at www.797-CompliancePro.com and can assist you in your efforts toward USP 797 compliance, so are recommended for you to utilize in addition to this book. Indeed, it is highly likely that the SOPs, form, logs, and templates provided in this educational program will be all that you actually need to generate the documentation required by regulatory entities inspecting your site for USP 797 compliance. Meanwhile, I do advise you to check at least annually for changes to state and federal regulations (such as those applicable to your state's Board of Pharmacy or the *FDA*) since these can – and do – periodically change. You may also want in future to re-read specific chapters in this book as so much information was packed into each chapter to make it a "fast read."

Congratulations, you have just read the last page in this book. It is now time to get started on utilizing the new knowledge you have gained to increase the likelihood that adherence to USP "best practices" is occurring at your health clinic, wellness center, or other business offering IV vitamin infusions!

ABOUT THE AUTHOR

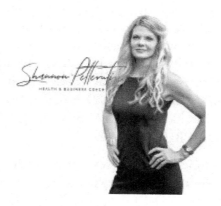

Shannon Petteruti is a serial entrepreneur, speaker, and health expert who has been featured in INC. Magazine, NBC, Thrive Global, PBN News, and Authority Magazine. She is best known for helping her clients live their most abundant lives through overcoming obstacles, finding their path, and reaching their goals.

Shannon has used her professional career to focus on helping others achieve their maximum health and has had several successful businesses focused on this mission. After graduating from Simmons College as a Sigma Theta Tau International Honors graduate with dual bachelor degrees in business management and nursing, she went on to become a board-certified nurse practitioner and earn a Master's degree in nursing. Shannon has now worked in the healthcare landscape for 20 years, using her education and passion to boost the success of her businesses.

For her first business venture, Shannon wanted to focus on birth, child development, and helping families so she launched Bellani Maternity out of her garage. Within the first year, Shannon was able to successfully grow her new business to $1 million in sales. Bellani Maternity went on to become an award-winning company with Shannon leading the way as CEO.

After six years in this role, Shannon transitioned from the leadership role to continue her education in anti-aging, functional medicine, IV vitamin therapy and USP 797 sterile compounding training as she wanted to pursue her growing passion for nursing and more patient-centered care. In 2014, this led to Shannon to take on the role of CEO of Intellectual Medicine, a concierge medical practice with a keen focus on personal health care. Shannon has proven her success, expertise and dedication to the personal health care industry in her past roles as CEO, and from 2019 – 2021 brought these tools to the table as CEO and co-founder of the award winning IV vitamin infusion business, THE DRIPBaR Franchise.

Through these business endeavors over the past 20 years, Shannon has also focused on the success of her clients. She has helped hundreds of men and women lose weight, achieve hormone balance, and lead healthy and vital lives.

You can find her at the following locations:

Website: www.ShannonPetteruti.com

Website: www.USP797compliancepro.com

Email: shannon@shannonpetteruti.com

facebook.com/ShannonPetteruti
twitter.com/PetterutiNP
instagram.com/ShannonPetteruti.NP
linkedin.com/in/shannonpetteruti

REFERENCES

Agalloco, J, Akers, J, Madsen, R. Aseptic Processing: A Review of Current Industry Practice. Pharmaceutical Technology. 2004: 28 (10, Oct):128.

ASTM D6978 - 05(2013) Standard practice for assessment of resistance of medical gloves to permeation by chemotherapy drugs, available for purchase at https://www.astm.org/Standards/D6978.htm. Accessed January 11, 2022

Center for Disease Control and Prevention, Multistate outbreak of fungal meningitis and other infections. https://www.cdc.gov/hai/outbreaks/meningitis.html. Accessed January 11, 2022

Center for Medicare and Medicaid Services. Site operations manual for hospitals and critical access hospitals, appendix a, survey protocol, regulations and interpretive guidelines for hospitals. https://www.cms.gov/Regulations-and-Guidance/Guidance/Manuals/downloads/som107ap_a_hospitals.pdf. Accessed January 11, 2022

Center for Medicare and Medicaid Services. Site operations manual for hospitals and critical access hospitals, appendix. w, survey protocol, regulations and interpretive guidelines for critical access hospitals

REFERENCES

(CAHs) and swing-beds in CAHs. https://www.cms.gov/Regulations-and-Guidance/Guidance/Manuals/downloads/som107ap_w_cah.pdf. Accessed January 10, 2022

Congress.gov. H.R.3204 — Drug Quality and Security Act. 113th Congress (2013–2014). https://www.congress.gov/bill/113th-congress/house-bill/3204. Accessed December 20, 2021

CriticalPoint: Home. Accessed February 27, 2022. https://www.criticalpoint.info/

Critical Point. The Brutal Facts About Compounding. Critical Point's Sterile Compounding Boot Camp™. Powerpoint presentation. Copyright 2013-2014.

Douglass, Kate, Kastango, Eric S, MBA RPh, Cantor, Peter. Let This Be Your Wake-up Call. Pharmacy Purchasing & Products. October 2014. http://www.pppmag.com/article/1588/October_2014_Cleanrooms_Compounding/Let_This_Be_Your_Wakeup_Call/?Kasst ango Accessed January 11, 2022

Eisler, Peter, Schnaars, Christopher. Safety, sanitary problems prompt many drug recalls. USA TODAY October 8, 2014.

General Chapter Pharmaceutical Compounding – Sterile Preparations. Usp.org. Published 2019. https://www.usp.org/compounding/general-chapter-797 Accessed February 27th, 2022.

General Questions about USP - SNMMI. www.snmmi.org. Accessed February 27, 2022. http://www.snmmi.org/IssuesAdvocacy/content.aspx?ItemNumber=4901

Guidance Document Compounding Record and Master Formulation Record for Sterile Compounds. http://www.ncbop.org/PDF/CompoundingRecordGuidanceDocumentUPDATED11_2017.pdf

Hawkins B, ASHP/BHH. *Drug Distribution and Control: Preparation and Handling–Guidelines Purpose.*; 2015. Accessed February 27, 2022. http://www.ashp.org/doclibrary/bestpractices/prepgdlcsp.aspx

Hellums M, Alverson SP, Monk-Tutor MR. Instruction on compounded sterile preparations at U.S. schools of pharmacy. AJHP. Volume 64, Nov 1, 2007: 2267-74.

The Joint Commission. About The Joint Commission. https://www.jointcommission.org/about_us/about_the_joint_commission_main.aspx. Accessed January 11, 2022

The Joint Commission. Requirements for the medication compounding certification, general responsibilities (mdcgr) chapter, standard MDCGR.01. https://www.jointcommission.org/assets/1/6/Medication_Compounding_v2.pdf. Accessed January 11, 2022

Kastango, Eric S, MBA, RPh, FASHP, Kramer, Nancy, RN, BSN, CRNI. The Top 10 Things You Need to Know About USP <797>. Infusion. May/June 2009.

Lester D. *Practical Guide to Contemporary Pharmacy Practice 4th edition.* Lippincott Williams & Wilkins; 2018.

Myers CE. History of sterile compounding in US hospitals, learning from the tragic lessons of the past. *Am J Health Syst Pharm.* 2013;70(16):1414-1427.

New Report Examines Updates to Compounding Pharmacy Law > National Conference of State Legislatures. www.ncsl.org. Accessed February 27, 2022. http://www.ncsl.org/blog/2014/06/06/new-report-examines-updates-to-compounding-pharmacy-law.aspx

Notice of intent to revise USP general chapter <797> pharmaceutical compounding—sterile preparations. http://www.usp.org/sites/default/files/usp_pdf/EN/USPNF/usp-gc-797-proposed-revisions-sep-2015.pdf. Accessed January 6, 2022

Pharmaceutical Compounding – Sterile Preparations. USP.org. Retrieved March 15, 2016: http://www.usp.org/sites/default/files/usp_pdf/EN/USPNF/usp-gc-797-proposed-revisions-sep-2015.pdf Accessed January 11, 2022

Pew Charitable Trust: U.S. Illnesses and Deaths Associated With Compounded Medications http://www.pewtrusts.org/en/about/news-

REFERENCES

room/news/2013/09/06/us-illnesses-and-deaths-associated-with-compoundedmedications Accessed January 11, 2022

Proper D and Johnson E. Non-Sterile Compounding for Pharmacy Technicians Training and Review for Certification. McGraw-Hill Education. 2015. EISBN 9780071829892

Proposed USP general chapter <797> pharmaceutical compounding—sterile preparations, September 2015. http://www.usp.org/sites/default/files/usp_pdf/EN/USPNF/usp-gc-797-proposed-revisions-sep-2015.pdf. Accessed January 11, 2022

Quality Standards at Empower Pharmacy. www.empowerpharmacy.com. Accessed February 27, 2022. https://www.empowerpharmacy.com/about/quality

Research C for DE and. Registered Outsourcing Facilities. *FDA*. Published online February 24, 2022. Accessed February 27, 2022. https://www.fda.gov/drugs/human-drug-compounding/registered-outsourcing-facilities

State of pharmacy compounding: <797> compliance. *Pharm Purch Prod*. April 2016, *www.pppmag.com. Accessed January 11, 2022

State Oversight of Compounding Pharmacies Varies Dramatically. American Pharmacists Association. Published February 25, 2016: https://www.pharmacist.com/state-oversight-compounding-pharmacies-varies-dramatically Accessed January 11, 2022

State Regulation of Compounding Pharmacies. National Conference of State Legislatures. Published October 1, 2014: http://www.ncsl.org/research/health/regulating-compounding-pharmacies.aspx Accessed January 11, 2022

Sterile Compounding Tragedy is a Symptom of a Broken System on Many Levels. Institute For Safe Medication Practices. Accessed February 27, 2022. http://www.ismp.org/newsletters/acutecare/showarticle.aspx?id=34

United States Pharmacopeial Convention, Inc. 795 Pharmaceutical Compounding-Nonsterile Preparations.

Made in the USA
Columbia, SC
22 June 2022